In Clinical Practice

Taking a practical approach to clinical medicine, this series of smaller reference books is designed for the trainee physician, primary care physician, nurse practitioner and other general medical professionals to understand each topic covered. The coverage is comprehensive but concise and is designed to act as a primary reference tool for subjects across the field of medicine.

Jean J. Filipov

Therapeutic Plasma Exchange

Current Trends in Clinical Practice

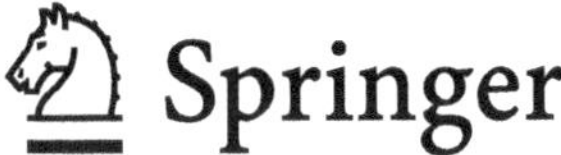

Jean J. Filipov
Department of Nephrology & Transplantation
Alexandrovska Hospital
Sofia, Bulgaria

ISSN 2199-6652 ISSN 2199-6660 (electronic)
In Clinical Practice
ISBN 978-3-032-17274-7 ISBN 978-3-032-17275-4 (eBook)
https://doi.org/10.1007/978-3-032-17275-4

This Springer imprint is published by the registered company Springer Nature Switzerland AG
The registered company address is: Gewerbestrasse 11, 6330 Cham, Switzerland

Preface

Therapeutic apheresis (TA) is a medical procedure in which plasma, blood cells, and blood-soluble molecules are separated from whole blood; the target component (plasma, blood cells, or blood-soluble molecule) is either removed or modified and returned to the patient. Therapeutic plasma exchange (PEX) is the most widely used form of TA, in which patient's plasma is separated from blood cells. Blood cells are pumped back into circulation, whereas patient's plasma is removed and is substituted by human albumin and/or fresh frozen plasma (FFP). Thus, large molecules, e.g., pathogenic immunoglobulins, are removed from the body. The therapeutic method was developed in the first half of the twentieth century, and significant improvement in effectiveness and patient safety has been observed over the years. In addition, the scope of PEX and its indications has been broadening constantly. However, PEX beneficial effect varies across different diseases.

The aim of this book is to present the basic principles of PEX, to demonstrate various alternatives of the procedure, and to depict the current data on its effectiveness and suggested PEX regimens in different clinical specialties.

Sofia, Bulgaria Jean J. Filipov

Acknowledgments

I would like to thank my family for the support throughout the writing of this book.

I would also like to thank my colleagues for their invaluable assistance in performing plasma exchange in our Department.

Competing Interests The author has no competing interests to declare that are relevant to the content of this manuscript.

Contents

About the Author

Jean J. Filipov graduated from the Medical University in Sofia in 2002. He obtained specialty in internal medicine (2010) and nephrology (2015). From December 2003 till November 2020 and from October 2021 to date, he worked at the Department of Nephrology and Transplantation, University Hospital Alexandrovska, Sofia, Bulgaria. He was head of the Dialysis Unit in the same hospital (December 2021–January 2023), as well as assistant professor in the Medical University–Sofia, Bulgaria (2005–2020). From December 2020 till October 2021, he was part of the renal and transplantation team in University Hospital Lozenetz, Sofia, Bulgaria. In 2015, he obtained his PhD degree with the topic of the doctoral thesis: "Vitamin D and kidney transplantation." Additionally, he has worked as specialist registrar at John Walls Renal Unit, Leicester, UK (November 2011–April 2012). Since 2013, he is involved in the plasma exchange program of the Department of Nephrology and Transplantation and was part of the team that developed the Plasma Exchange Guidelines for the Bulgarian Society of Nephrology in 2016. Except for plasma exchange, he is professionally interested in mineral bone disease in chronic kidney disease, onconephrology, and kidney transplantation.

Abbreviations

AAV	ANCA-associated vasculitis
AB0i	AB0 incompatible
AbMR	Antibody-mediated rejection
ACD	Anticoagulant citrate dextrose solution
ACE	Angiotensin converting enzyme
ACLF	Acute-on-chronic liver failure
ACP	Adsorptive cytapheresis
ACR	Cellular acute rejection
ACS	Acute chest syndrome
ADAMTS13	A disintegrin and metalloproteinase with a thrombospondin type 1 motif, member 13
ADEM	Acute disseminated encephalomyelitis
AHA	Autoimmune hemolytic anemia
AKI	Acute kidney injury
AlAT	Alanine aminotransferase
ALF	Acute liver failure
ALL	Acute lymphoblastic leukemia
AML	Acute myeloid leukemia
ANCA	Antineutrophil cytoplasmic antibody
anti-MPO	Autoantibodies anti myeloperoxidase antibodies
anti-PLA2R-Ab	Anti-phospholipase A2 receptor antibodies
anti-PR3	Antibodies anti-protein 3 antibodies
APCS	Alternative pathway of the complement system
ApoB	Apolipoprotein B

ApolB100	Apolipoprotein B100
APS	Antiphospholipid syndrome
aPTT	Activated partial thromboplastin time
AR	Acute rejection
ARB	Angiotensin receptor blockers
AsAT	Aspartate aminotransferase
ASFA	Amerucan Society for Apheresis
AT	Antithrombin
ATG	Anti-thymocyte globulin
AVF	Arteriovenous fistula
AVG	Arteriovenous graft
BW	Body weight
CAPS	Catastrophic antiphospholipid syndrome
CD	Crohn's disease
cGVHD	Chronic graft versus host disease
CIDP	Chronic inflammatory demyelinating polyradiculoneuropathy
CKD	Chronic kidney disease
CLL	Chronic lymphocytic leukemia
cmTMA	Complement-mediated thrombotic microangiopathy
CMV	Cytomegalovirus
CNI	Calcineurin inhibitor
CNS	Central nervous system
cPEX	Centrifugal therapeutic plasma exchange
CPP	Cryo-precipitate poor plasma
CRRT	Continuous renal replacement therapy
CS	Corticosteroids
CSF	Cerebrospinal fluid
CT	Computer tomography
CVC	Central venous catheter
CVD	Cardiovascular disease
CVVH	Continuous venovenous hemofiltration
CYC	Cyclophosphamide
D	Daltons
DAH	Diffuse alveolar hemorrhage
DALI	Direct adsorption of lipoproteins
DFPP	Double filtration plasmapheresis

DIC	Disseminated intravascular coagulopathy
diTMA	Drug-induced thrombotic microangiopathy
DN-PEX	Double needle PEX
DOAC	Direct oral anticoagulant
DSA	Donor-specific antibodies
DSA-HLA	Donor-specific anti-HLA antibodies
EBV	Epstein-Barr virus
ECP	Extracorporeal photopheresis
EGP	Eosinophilic granulomatosis with polyangiitis
EPV	Estimated plasma volume
FFP	Fresh frozen plasma
FH	Familial hypercholesterolemia
Fibr	Fibrinogen
FLC	Free light chains
FPSA	Fractionated Plasma Separation and Adsorption System
FSGS	Focal segmental glomerulosclerosis
GBM	Glomerular basement membrane
GBS	Guillain-Barré syndrome
GMP	Granulomatosis with polyangiitis
GVHD	Graft versus host disease
HA	Hemoadsorption
HbS	Hemoglobin S
HBV	Hepatitis B
HCV	Hepatitis C
HeFH	Heterozygous familial hypercholesterolemia
HELLP	Hemolysis, Elevated Liver enzymes, Low Platelet count
HELP	Heparin-induced extracorporeal precipitation
HIV	Human immunodefficiency virus
HLAP	Hyperlipidemic acute pancreatitis
HoFH	Homozygous familial hypercholesterolemia
HSCT	Hematopoietic stem cell transplantation
HT	Heart transplantation
HV-PEX	High volume PEX
HVS	Hyperviscosity syndrome
IA	Immunoadsorption
IAGD	Infection-associated glomerular disease

iaTMA	Infection associated TMA
IBD	Inflammatory bowel disease
iCa	Ionized calcium
ICI	Immune check-point inhibitors
IDCM	Idiopathic dilated cardiomyopathy
Ig	Immunoglobulin
IgAN	IgA nephropathy
IgAV	IgA vasculitis
INR	International normalized ratio
IV	Intravenous
IVIG	Intravenous immunoglobulins
kD	Kilodaltons
KT	Kidney transplantation
LA	Lipoprotein apheresis
LCA	Leukocytapheresis
LDH	Lactate dehydrogenase
LDL	Low-density lipoproteins
LEMS	Lambert Eaton myasthenic syndrome
LMH	Low molecular heparin
LN	Lupus nephritis
LPRP4	Lipoprotein-related protein 4
LT	Liver transplantation
MARS	Molecular adsorbent circulating system
MCD	Minimal change disease
MF	Mycosis fungoides
MFI	Mean fluorescence intensity
MG	Myasthenia gravis
MGCS	Monoclonal gammopathy of clinical significance
MGUS	Monoclonal gammopathy of undetermined significance
MM	Multiple myeloma
MN	Membranous nephropathy
MOF	Multiorgan failure
MOG	Myelin oligodendrocyte glycoprotein
MPA	Microscopoic polyangiitis
mPEX	Membrane therapeutic plasma exchange
MPGN	Membranoproliferative glomerulonephritis

MRI	Magnetic resonance imaging
MS	Multiple sclerosis
mTMA	Malignancy-associated thrombotic microangiopathy
mTORi	Mammalian target of Rapamycin inhibitors
MUSK	Muscle-specific kinase
MW	Molecular weight
nACHR	Nicotinic acetylcholine receptor
Neu	Neutrophils
NMDARA	N-Methyl-D-Aspartate Receptor Antibody
NMOSD	Neuromyelitis optica spectrum disorder
NSAIDs	Nonsteroidal anti-inflammatory drugs
PAD	Peripheral artery disease
PAN	Polyarteritis nodosa
PANi	Idiopathic polyarteritis nodosa
PCSK9	Proprotein convertase subtilisin/kexin 9
PE	Pre-eclampsia
PE-SF	Pre-eclampsia severe form
PEX	Therapeutic plasma exchange
PICC	Peripherally inserted central catheters
PLT	Platelets
PNPS	Paraneoplastic syndromes
PRCA	Pure red cell aplasia
pTMA	Pregnancy-associated thrombotic microangiopathy
PV	Polycytemia vera
Qbf	Blood flow in a single hollow fiber
Qbt	Total blood flow of the separator
Qf	Filtration flow
RBC	Red blood cells
RPGN	Rapidly progressive glomerulonephritis
RRT	Renal replacement therapy
RTX	Rituximab
SCD	Sickle cell disease
SLE	Systemic lupus erythematosus
SN	PEX single needle PEX
SOFA	Sepsis-related organ failure assessment
SOT	Solid organ transplantation

SPAD	Single pass albumin dialysis
SRC	Scleroderma renal crisis
SS	Sézary syndrome
SSC	Systemic sclerosis
St-EC	Shiga-like toxin producing strains of E.coli
T3	Triiodothyronine
T4	Thyroxine
TA	Therapeutic apheresis
T-AHG	Antiglobulin T-cell cross match test
TA-TMA	Transplantation-associated thrombotic micro-angiopathy
TBV	Total blood volume
TCA	Thrombocytapheresis
tCVC	Tunneled central venous catheters
TLS	Tumor lysis syndrome
TMA	Thrombotic Microangiopathy
TMP	Transmembrane pressure
TPEX/HD	Tandem PEX and hemodialysis
TSH	Thyroid stimulating hormone
TTP	Thrombotic thrombocytopenic purpura
UC	Ulcerative colitis
UFH	Unfractionated heparin
Vd	Volume of distribution
VGPCD	Voltage-gated potassium channel antibody disorders
VLDL	Very low density lipoproteins
VP	Venous ports
vWF	Von Willebrand factor
WBC	White blood cells
WD	Wilson disease

1 Introduction. History of Plasma Exchange. Definition of Terms

Abstract

Plasma separation techniques were tested more than a century ago, firstly in animal models, later they were introduced in human medicine. The advance of separation techniques led to broadening of the therapeutic indications and improving patient's safety. This chapter briefly outlines the history of therapeutic apheresis (TA) and plasma exchange. The most important definitions used in apheresis today are presented.

Keywords

Therapeutic apheresis · Plasmapheresis · Cytapheresis · History of apheresis · Definitions

History of Plasma Exchange

Bloodletting is a procedure known since antiquity. However, the first attempts for separation of plasma from blood cells were performed at the beginning of twentieth century. In 1913, Yurevich and Rosenberg effused limited volume of blood, which was substituted simultaneously with saline in rabbits. The blood was centrifuged, plasma platelets and white blood cells were removed,

J. J. Filipov, *Therapeutic Plasma Exchange*, In Clinical Practice,
https://doi.org/10.1007/978-3-032-17275-4_1

whereas red blood cells were washed out several times. The main idea was to evaluate the possibility of extracorporeal removal of toxins. All experimental animals tolerated the procedure well [1]. In 1914, Abel successfully removed plasma from blood in dogs, with return of the blood cells by centrifugation, a process he called for the first time *plasmapheresis* [2].

The first plasma removal in humans was performed in 1926 by Gilbert et al. [3]. In 1944, Tui et al. used centrifugal plasmapheresis to obtain plasma for donation in humans [4]. Gradually the use of the procedure expanded further as a treatment option—first in the treatment of multiple myeloma [5]. In 1976, membrane separation technique was introduced, whereas in early 1980s, selective separation procedures were demonstrated—immunoadsorption, cascade filtration, cryofiltration, thermofiltration, and LDL adsorption [6]. These new options enabled the physicians to remove selective plasma components without loss of vital substances, thus increasing therapeutic effectiveness and improving patient safety.

Definition of Terms

Translated from Greek, apheresis means removal, taking away. In order to avoid confusions, the basic terms were introduced in 1983 by the International Society of Artificial Organs.

Apheresis

In modern medicine, apheresis is a procedure, in which one or more blood components are separated from whole blood and are removed. In therapeutic apheresis (TA), removed components (plasma, blood cells, and blood-soluble molecules) are either substituted or returned to the patient after modification (e.g., adsorption, cryofiltration, and cascade filtration) [7]. Therapeutic apheresis and its relation to other extracorporeal blood purification methods are demonstrated in Fig. 1.1.

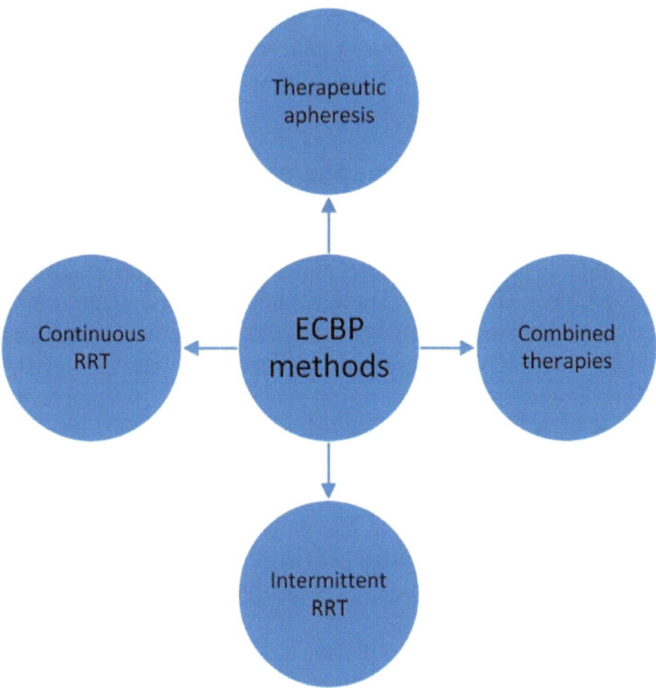

Fig. 1.1 Therapeutic apheresis and other extracorporeal blood purification methods. *ECBP*extracorporeal blood purification, *RRT* renal replacement therapy

Plasmapheresis and Therapeutic Plasma Exchange

Generally, plasmapheresis means separation and removal of plasma from blood. The procedure is widely applied in preparation of transfusion components from healthy donors. Donation plasmapheresis usually is limited to 500 ml [7]; donation plasmapheresis will not be discussed in this book.

Therapeutic plasmapheresis refers to the procedure in which plasma is separated from whole blood and is either discarded, coupled with adequate substitution fluid (FFP, albumin), or is modified and then returned to the patient, without substitution.

Therapeutic plasma exchange signifies the process of separation and removal of plasma in patients; the removed plasma is substituted with FFP or albumin solution.

Double Filtration Plasmapheresis

This refers to the process of separating plasma from whole blood via filtration and subsequent second filtration of already separated plasma. In standard PEX, abnormal plasma is discarded, leading to protein loss and risk for bleeding. Therefore, techniques processing the initially filtered plasma were created. Once plasma has been separated from blood by specific filter, it undergoes additional filtration (using a second or even third filter) and is returned to the patient. The following are the major options:

- Cryofiltration—separated plasma is cooled in order to microaggregates to be formed, which in turn are removed by second filtration. After warming, the twice-filtered plasma is returned to the patient.
- Thermofiltration—after plasma is separated, it is warmed up, so that certain molecules (LDL, VLDL) form aggregates. The plasma is filtered again and is returned to patient's circulation.
- Double filtration plasmapheresis or Cascade filtration—separated plasma is being filtered several more times so that certain plasma molecules are filtered and returned to the patient; the rest of the plasma is discarded.

Plasma Adsorption and Hemoadsorption

In plasma adsorption, pathogenic molecules are removed by adhering to a sorbent (adsorption). Plasma is initially separated from whole blood and runs through adsorbent and is returned to the patient. Three major subtypes are present:

- Unselective plasma adsorption—plasma runs through unselective adsorbent, e.g., charcoal or ion exchange resins.
- Selective plasma adsorption—separated plasma runs through nonimmune adsorbent molecules (e.g., dextran sulfate in LDL adsorption).
- Immunoadsorption—the adsorbent molecules are specific antigens or antibodies, thus removing specific antibodies/antigens in the treated plasma.

If whole blood runs through adsorbent, the process is called *hemoadsorption.*

Selective plasma adsorption techniques, especially immunoadsorption, will be discussed in the following chapters.

Apheresis of Blood Cells (Cytapheresis)

Cytapheresis is the removal of blood cells from blood. Therapeutic cytapheresis targets a certain pathologic cell type in oncology/hematology. Several types are present:

- Erythrocytapheresis—removal of red blood cells (RBC) from blood. When erythrocytapheresis is coupled with infusion of RBC concentrate, the procedure is called RBC exchange.
- Thrombocytapheresis—removal of platelets as therapeutic option or donation.
- Leukocytapheresis (or leukapheresis)—nonselective removal of white blood cells.
- Granulocytapheresis—selective removal of granulocytes.
- Lymphocytapheresis—selective removal of lymphocytes.

These methods will be discussed in other sections of this book. Figure 1.2 summarizes the major types of therapeutic apheresis.

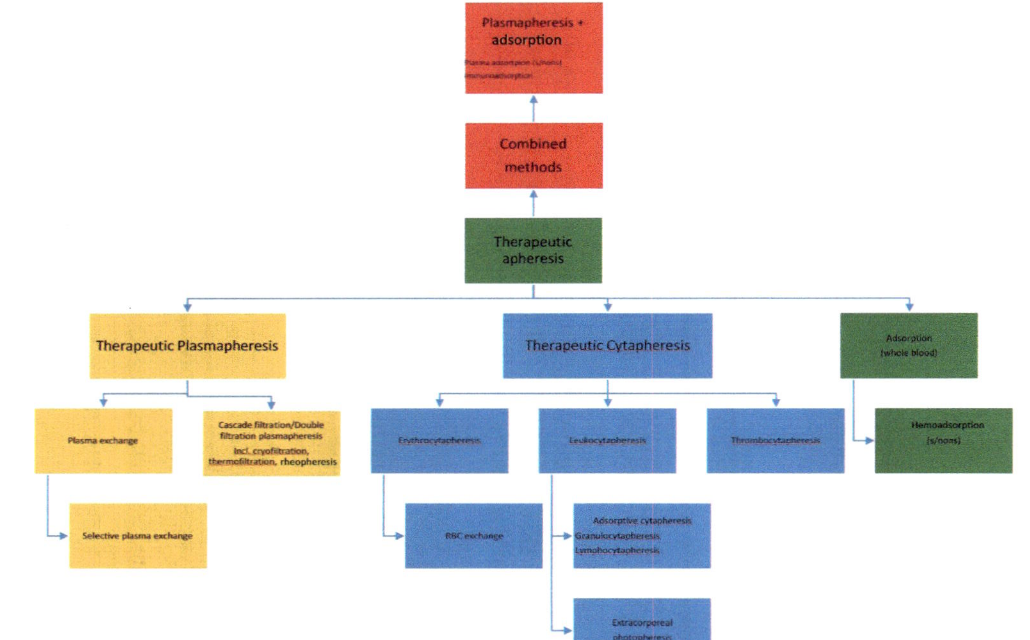

Fig. 1.2 Major types of therapeutic apheresis

References

1. Sokolov AA, Solovyev AG. Russian pioneers of therapeutic hemapheresis and extracorporeal hemocorrection: 100-year anniversary of the world's first successful plasmapheresis. Ther Apher Dial. 2014;18(2):117–21. https://doi.org/10.1111/1744-9987.12067.
2. Clark WF, Huang SS. Introduction to therapeutic plasma exchange. Transfus Apher Sci. 2019;58(3):228–9. https://doi.org/10.1016/j.transci.2019.04.004.
3. Stegmayr BG. A survey of blood purification techniques. Transfus Apher Sci. 2005;32(2):209–20. https://doi.org/10.1016/j.transci.2004.10.023.
4. Tui C, Bartter FC, Wright AM, Holt RB. Red cell reinfusion and the frequency of plasma donations: preliminary report of multiple donations in eight weeks by each of six donors. JAMA. 1944;124(6):331–6. https://doi.org/10.1001/jama.1944.02850060001001.
5. Judson G, Jones A, Kellogg R, Buckner D, Eisel R, Perry S, et al. Closed continuous-flow centrifuge. Nature. 1968;217:816–8. https://doi.org/10.1038/217816a0.
6. Bambauer R, Latza R, Schiel R. Introduction. In: Therapeutic plasma exchange and selective plasma separation methods: fundamental technologies, pathophysiology, and clinical results. 4th ed. Lengerich: Pabst Science Publisher; 2013. p. 35–50.
7. Ostermann M, Ankawi G, Cantaluppi V, Madarasu R, Dolan K, Husain-Syed F, et al. Nomenclature of extracorporeal blood purification therapies for acute indications: the nomenclature standardization conference. Blood Purif. 2024;53:358–72. https://doi.org/10.1159/000533468.

2 Principles of Therapeutic Plasma Exchange

Abstract

In this chapter, the basic principles of therapeutic plasma exchange will be discussed—plasma separation techniques, mechanism of action of PEX, substitution solutions, anticoagulation, vascular access, concomitant immunosuppression, and possible complications of the procedure. More selective alternatives for PEX will be reviewed, as well as methods for cytapheresis.

Keywords

Plasma separation · Selective techniques · Vascular access · PEX prescription · Adverse events

Plasma Separation

In therapeutic plasma exchange (PEX), patient's blood is pumped out of the body and is transferred to plasma separator that removes plasma from whole blood. In the standard PEX procedure, separated plasma is discarded, whereas blood cells are pumped back into patient's circulation. Patient's plasma is substituted by human albumin solutions or FFP, which is infused into the blood cells after plasma separation, prior to pumping back blood cells into the patient. Figure 2.1 demonstrates schematically a standard

J. J. Filipov, *Therapeutic Plasma Exchange*, In Clinical Practice,
https://doi.org/10.1007/978-3-032-17275-4_2

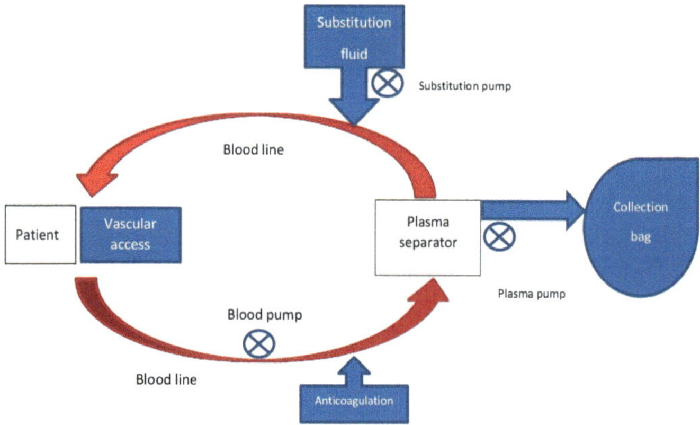

Fig. 2.1 Diagram of therapeutic plasma exchange

plasma exchange procedure. The procedure is performed by computerized devices. Photo 2.1 demonstrates plasma exchange (membrane separator).

Note: anticoagulation with low molecular heparin (LMH) is administered as a single dose at the beginning of plasma exchange.

There are two types of plasma separation methods—centrifugal and membrane separation.

Centrifugal Plasma Separation

The plasma separator is a bowl, which removes plasma from blood by centrifugation at the speed of 2000–2500 revolutions per minute. By centrifugation, other blood components are also being separated, e.g., platelets, white blood cells, and red blood cells—Fig. 2.2.

Centrifugal PEX (cPEX) can remove all types of protein molecules; red blood cells are returned into patient's circulation either simultaneously or intermittently. Apart from removing all protein fractions, cPEX has a major advantage that peripheral vein can be used as vascular access, compared to membrane PEX. In cPEX,

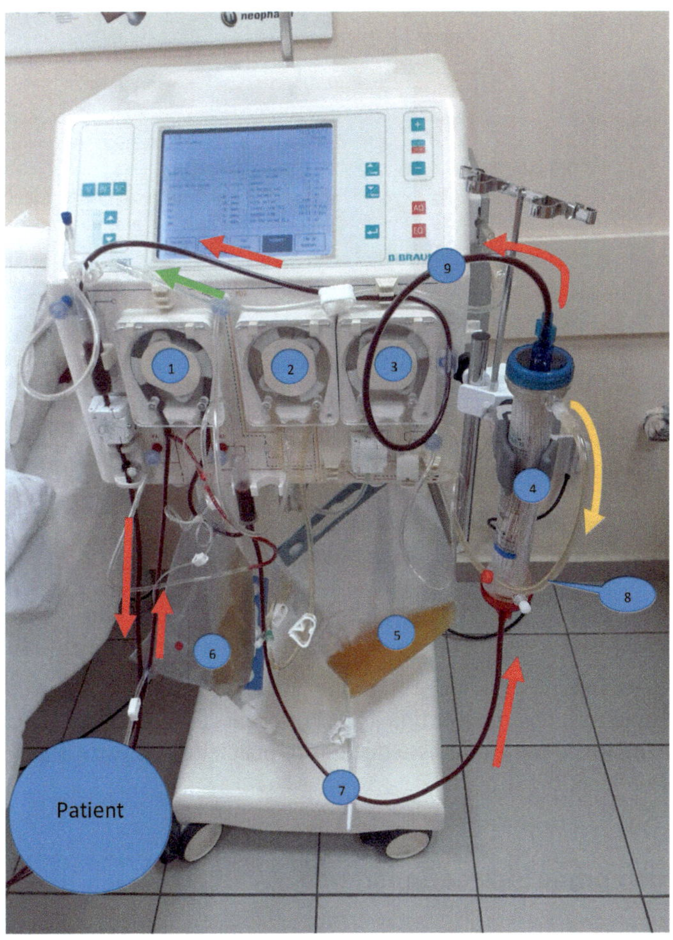

Photo 2.1 Plasma exchange with membrane separator (Diapact® CRRT machine, B. Braun Avitum AG, Germany). (1) Blood pump; (2) Plasma pump; (3) Substitution pump; (4) Membrane plasma separator; (5) Effluent collection bag; (6) Substitution fluid; (7) Blood line (arterial, blood from patient); (8) Plasma outlet line, (9) Blood line (venous, blood returning to the patient); red arrow—blood flow; yellow arrow—plasma effluent flow; green arrow—substitution fluid flow

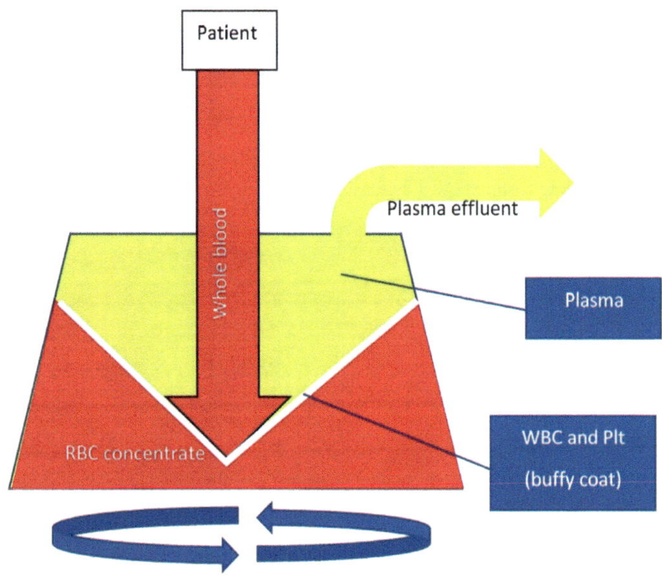

Fig. 2.2 Plasma separation by centrifugation

larger plasma percentage from the processed plasma is removed (up to 80%) per unit of time and shorter procedures are possible. A major complication is reduction in platelet count, which may drop by 50% [1, 2].

Membrane Plasma Separation

Membrane plasma separation currently is performed via hollow-fiber membrane separators. Similarly to hemodialysis, patient's blood runs through the hollow fibers of the separator and plasma is filtered through the pores of the semipermeable membrane—Fig. 2.3. Photo 2.2 demonstrates plasma filter during PEX. Blood cells are returned simultaneously. However, the driving force for plasma removal is convection, with primary factors being trans-

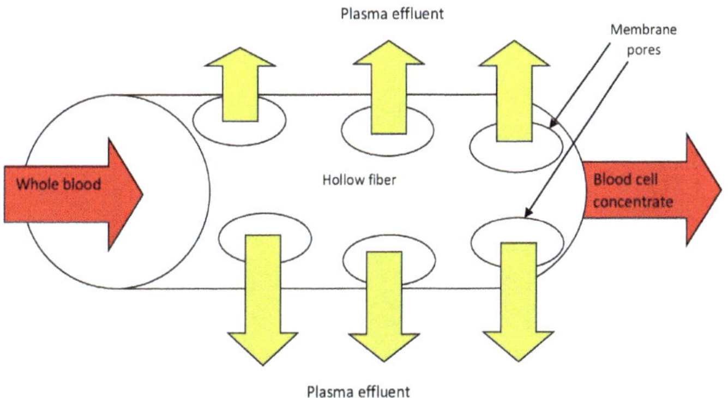

Fig. 2.3 Hollow-fiber membrane plasma separation

membrane pressure and membrane characteristics. Blood cells are returned simultaneously in the circulation. Currently devices for other continuous renal replacement therapy (CRRT) methods can be used for membrane therapeutic plasma exchange (mPEX) too.

Membrane plasma filter structure Modern membrane filters consists of a plastic cylinder, in which a large number of hollow fibers are inserted. The hollow fibers consist of semipermeable membrane—Photo 2.3.

Most plasma filters have total effective membrane surface ranging between 0.5 and 0.7 m^2. The number of hollow fibers within the filter varies between 700 and 2100. Their effective length varies from 115 to 230 mm, fibers' internal diameter ranges from 215 to 330 μm, and membrane thickness is in the range of 60–100 μm. Blood pump speed should not exceed 200 ml/min in order to avoid hemolysis; it is generally recommended filters not to be reused [2, 3].

Ideally, membranes and hollow fibers should possess the following properties: adequate pore radius, high porosity (high number of pores), small tortuosity, high diffusion coefficient, small protein adsorption on membrane surface, and thin active membrane layer to provide good permeability [4].

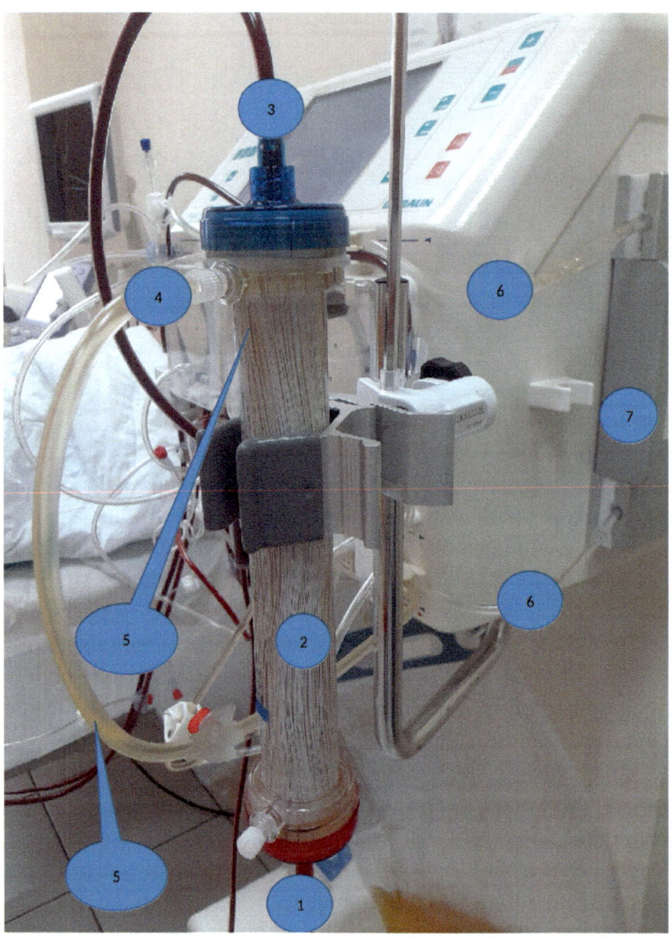

Photo 2.2 Plasma filter with filtered plasma during plasma exchange. (1) Filter inlet and arterial line; (2) Hollow fibers; (3) Filter outlet, and venous line; (4) Filtrate outlet; (5) Plasma effluent; (6) Substitution fluid; (7) Plate heater for substitution fluid (Haemoselect®, B. Braun Avitum AG, Germany)

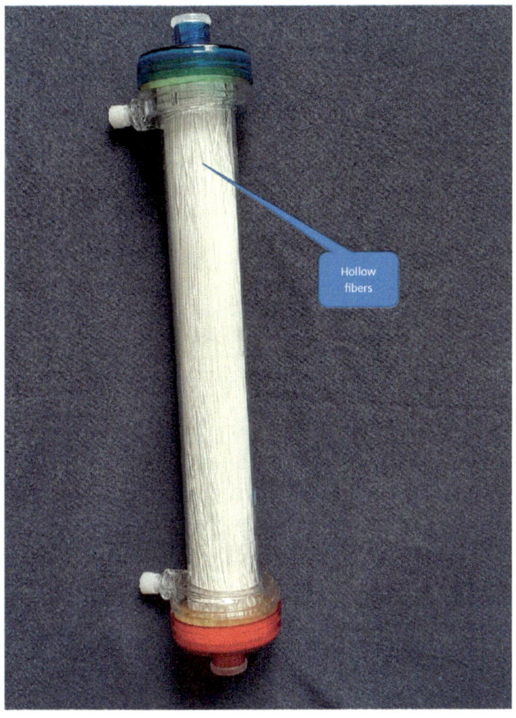

Photo 2.3 Membrane plasma separator with hollow fibers. (Haemoselect®, B. Braun Avitum AG, Germany)

In membrane plasma separation, larger membrane pores are used, with diameter of 0.2–0.5 μm, in contrast to 0.002–0.004 μm pore diameter in hemodialysis. This diameter has proved to provide the optimal filtrate speed, with lower risk for hemolysis [3]. Thus large molecules with high molecular mass (e.g., albumin, immunoglobulins) are removed by filtration into the inter-fiber space—Fig. 2.4.

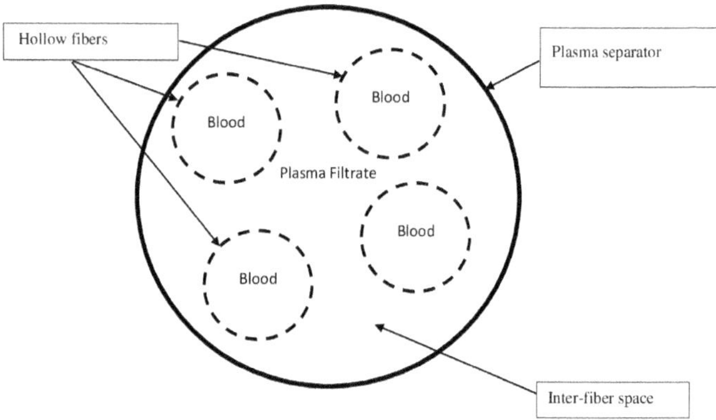

Fig. 2.4 Diagram of the membrane plasma separator

Membrane composition Different membrane materials are used. The major types are listed below:

- Cellulose diacetate.
- Polyvinyl alcohol.
- Polycarbonate.
- Polypropylene.
- Polyethylene.
- Polyethersulfone.

Filter membranes have asymmetrical structure—thin active membrane layer on the blood side with thickness of 1 μm and a thicker porous structure from the same material, supporting the active inner layer.

Two parameters characterize the different membrane materials:

Biocompatibility is currently defined as the ability of a material to perform its desired functions with respect to a medical therapy, to induce an appropriate host response in a specific application, and to interact with living systems without having any risk of injury, toxicity, or rejection by the immune system and undesirable or inappropriate local or systemic effects [5]. Membrane biocompatibility was previously defined by Brück as no thrombosis formation, no destruction of blood cells, no change in plasma proteins, including enzymes, no influencing of immune cells, as well as no damage for other organs and tissues [6].

Current use of polymers in membrane production for dialysis and plasma exchange led to improved biocompatibility and less side effects, compared to older membrane types (e.g., cellulose diacetate), mainly due to reduced immunoreactivity [7].

Sieving coefficient is defined as the ratio of filtrate concentration of a given substance to its blood concentration. A simple formula, describing sieving coefficient of a substance is presented in Eq. 2.1 [3]:

$$S = \frac{Cf}{\text{Cprefilter}} \tag{2.1}$$

S—sieving coefficient, *Cf*—filtrate concentration of the substance, Cprefilter—blood concentration of the substance before entering the filter.

A more complex formula is preferred in membrane plasma separation to calculate sieving coefficient, Eq. 2.2 [8]:

$$S = \frac{2Cf}{\text{Cprefilter} + \text{Cpostfilter}} \tag{2.2}$$

S—sieving coefficient, *Cf*—concentration of substance in filtrate, Cprefilter—concentration of substance prior to entering the filter, Cpostfilter—concentration of substance in the outlet of the filter.

Studies have demonstrated that polypropylene and polycarbonate membranes have higher sieving coefficient for IgA, IgG, and IgM molecules, compared to cellulose diacetate, as well as better filtrate flow, reflecting improvement in membrane technology [3]. Polypropylene and polyethylene achieved similar sieving coefficients for IgG, IgA, IgM, and albumin [9].

Improved characteristics of membranes led to optimized plasma protein removal as well as improved biocompatibility. Thus, currently, synthetic membrane filters are widely used. Hydrophilic membranes are recommended [10]. Principally, membrane type depends on the producer of the kit and the device for mPEX, available in the institution. In our institution, polyether sulfone membranes are available for mPEX (Haemoselect®, B. Braun Avitum AG, Germany), with an in vitro sieving coefficient for IgM and albumin of approx. 1. It should be mentioned that novel filters are being developed and are introduced into clinical practice, aiming for better efficiency and better safety profile [11].

Filtration flow In mPEX, pathogenic macromolecules are separated from blood by filtration. Therefore adequate filtration flow is required throughout the procedure for successful removal of plasma proteins. Filtration rate is influenced by the already mentioned characteristics of the membrane—high porosity, low tortuosity, thin active layer, high diffusion capacity, and adequate pore size. However, Jaffin et al. demonstrated that filtration flow (*Qf*) is correlated to membrane surface, wall shear rate, and quantity of fibers, whereas it is inversely related to effective length of the fibers [12].

Wall shear rate is defined as the change of velocity in the flow of fluid layers over the radius of a vessel or the hollow fiber. Wall shear rate is calculated by using the following formula Eq. 2.3, Fig. 2.5:

R—radius of hollow fiber, *V1*—velocity of blood flow at the wall of the fiber, *V2*—velocity of blood in the center of the fiber

$$\gamma = \frac{V1 - V2}{R} \tag{2.3}$$

γ—wall shear rate, *V1*—velocity of blood in the center of hollow fiber, *V2*—velocity of blood at the wall of hollow fiber, *R*—radius of hollow fiber.

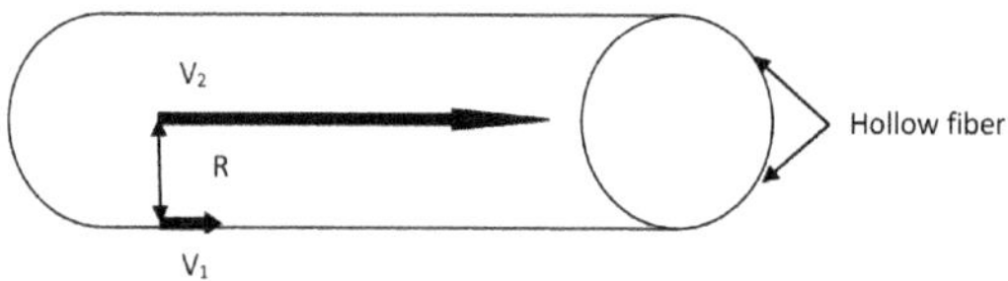

Fig. 2.5 Wall shear rate—diagram

As $V_2 = 0$, practically wall shear rate is—Eq. 2.4:

$$\gamma = \frac{V1}{R} \tag{2.4}$$

Shear rate γ is directly correlated to $V1$ and the blood flow within a single hollow fiber (*Qbf*) Eq.2.5:

$$\gamma = \frac{V1}{R} = \frac{4Qbf}{\pi R^3} \tag{2.5}$$

The sum of *Qbf* of all fibers within the separator equals the total blood flow (*Qbt*) Eq.6:

$$Qbt = N * Qbf \tag{2.6}$$

Qbt—total blood flow of the separator, *Qbf*—single fiber blood flow, *N*—number of fibers.

Wall shear rate is dependent on blood flow in the hollow fiber, which in turn is dependent on total blood flow in the separator, determined by the blood pump. Smaller fiber radius also increases shear rate.

In mPEX, the speed of blood flow rate is limited up to 200 ml/min due to the risk of hemolysis. In addition, blood flow higher than 200 ml/min does not increase filtration [2]. Practically, it rarely exceeds 150 ml/min. The lowest cut-off value for blood flow rate in mPEX demonstrated in the literature was 50 ml/min [13]. However, very low blood flow is also not recommended due to increased risk for filter clotting. Approximately 30% of the processed plasma are filtered per unit of time [1]. Thus, plasma pump (removing filtered plasma) and substitution pump (infusing substitution solution) speeds are limited to 30% of blood pump rate—Fig. 2.1. In our institution, blood flow rate for mPEX is within the range of 90–150 ml/min.

Transmembrane pressure (TMP) Transmembrane pressure (*TMP*) is defined as the pressure gradient between two sides of a membrane, in mPEX—between blood and filtered plasma on both sides of the hollow fiber. TMP is calculated by using the following equation—Eq. 2.7 [3]:

$$TMP = \frac{Pi + Po}{2} - Pf \tag{2.7}$$

TMP—transmembrane pressure; *Pi*—pressure in the inlet of the filter, depicted as PBE (blood entry pressure) in some dialysis machines; *Po*—pressure in the outlet of the filter, equivalent to *PV* (venous pressure) in some dialysis machines; *Pf*—pressure on the filtrate side, corresponds to *PD*2 in some dialysis machines—Photo 2.4a, b.

TMP is related to blood flow, membrane permeability, and hydrostatic and oncotic pressures across the membrane. Rise in TMP could theoretically increase filtration flow; however, increased TMP may cause hemolysis in mPEX and may cause membrane dysfunction. In addition, it has been demonstrated that TMP above 80 mmHg does not increase filtration [10]. Therefore, TMP should be kept as low as possible throughout the procedure. Current devices allow constant TMP monitoring during mPEX.

Generally, a rise in TMP is associated with clogging, clotting, and vascular access dysfunction. Clogging is the process of deposition of proteins along the semipermeable membrane. It causes gradual increase of TMP and membrane dysfunction. Clotting is the process of formation of blood clots within the hollow fibers, thus reducing the effective membrane surface, and is associated with a progressive or sudden rise in TMP. Vascular access dysfunction can cause rapid peak or drop in TMP [14, 15]. Inadequate vascular access can cause poor blood flow, leading to frequent interruptions of the procedure. This in turn increases the risk for clotting of the hollow fibers. Adequate anticoagulation, higher blood flow, and prefilter can be used to prevent clotting. Increase in blood flow may reduce filter clogging too [15].

Filter failure Filter failure during mPEX occurs as proteins and cells are deposited along the membrane, thus blocking its pores and forming a secondary membrane, which reduces effective blood flow and plasma filtration in the hollow fiber and finally compromising the procedure. The thickness of the secondary membrane increases from the inlet to the outlet of the separator. Clotting causes filter failure.

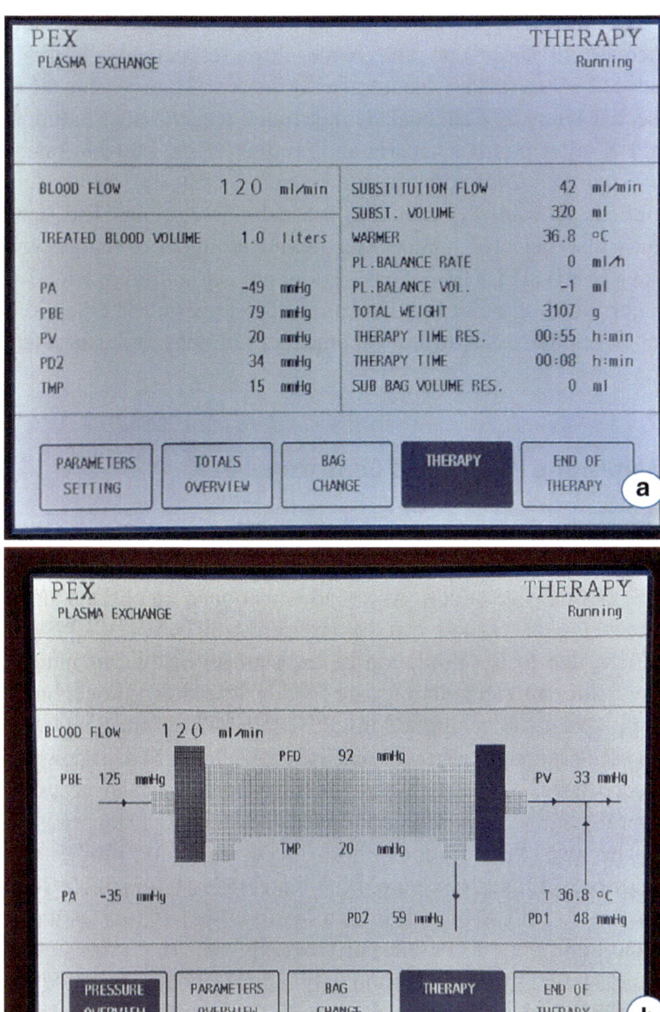

Photos 2.4 (**a**, **b**). Pressure data during membrane therapeutic plasma exchange (mPEX). *PBE* blood entry pressure, *PV* venous pressure, *TMP* transmembrane pressure, *PD*1 filter inlet pressure (filter inlet is blocked in mPEX), *PD*2 filter outlet pressure, *PA* pre-pump pressure in the arterial line, generated by the blood pump (always negative value). Different pressure presentations on monitor. (Diapact® CRRT machine, B. Braun Avitum AG, Germany)

Several strategies to avoid filter failure were suggested. Increase in shear rate and blood flow, respectively, partially reduced in secondary membrane formation [3]. A recent retrospective study by Elali et al. demonstrated reduced filter failure in mPEX, after prefilter heparin and prefilter saline infusion (mean infusion rate 241 ml/h, in the range of 200–400 ml/h) were applied, probably by reducing the risk for clotting. The same study also detected higher filter failure in higher exchange volumes (≥3 l) [16]. These measures did not cause fluid overload or major bleeding episodes. Therefore, the suggested interventions can be applied easily in clinical practice, without significant safety concerns.

Membrane PEX Versus Centrifugal PEX

The two modalities for PEX differ in their mechanisms for plasma separation which determines the differences in their performances and possible side effects. As already mentioned, in cPEX a larger percentage of plasma can be removed—80% vs. 30–35% in mPEX, due to the limitation of the semipermeable membrane. Thus, shorter treatment times are needed. In addition, lower blood pump speed can be applied in cPEX (50–150 ml/min), allowing the use of larger peripheral veins; in mPEX, higher blood rates are needed (90–200 ml/min), necessitating larger vascular access—central venous catheter or arteriovenous fistula [1, 13].

The two PEX options differ in their safety profile too. Centrifugal PEX is associated with increased risk for platelet loss, whereas in mPEX hemolysis can be observed, as well as membrane failure due to clotting or clogging [13]. However, studies demonstrated similar reduction in IgG, IgM, and fibrinogen levels in mPEX and cPEX, though in mPEX due to the presence of semipermeable membrane the removal of molecules larger than 30,000 daltons is restricted [2, 17]. Plasma removal efficacy will be discussed later in this chapter. Both cPEX and mPEX are used in pediatric patients, with similar benefit [18, 19]. A recent retrospective study demonstrated that mPEX was preferred in younger children (4.8 ± 2.8 years for mPEX vs. 15.2 ± 3.7 years for cPEX, $p = 0.0001$) and in children with lower body weight (19.5 ± 10.6 kg for mPEX vs. 71.7 ± 28.5 kg for cPEX, $P = 0.0001$), with similar safety profile between the two PEX modalities [20]. Membrane PEX has advantage over cPEX in younger children probably due to the smaller volume of extracorporeal circuit required in patients with lower body size (100–185 ml in cPEX vs. 65–94 ml in mPEX) [21]. It has been demonstrated that cPEX is associated with less circuit clotting [13, 20]. However, most of the devices for CRRT can perform mPEX. Thus, a single machine can be used for different therapeutic modalities, whereas cPEX requires specific device for the procedure. Table 2.1 summarizes the differences between cPEX and mPEX.

Table 2.1 Parameters of centrifugal and membrane plasma exchange [1, 2, 13, 20, 21]

Parameter	Centrifugal PEX	Membrane PEX
Mechanism of plasma separation	Centrifugation	Convection
Large molecules removal **Lower limit** (MW)	>15,000 D	>15,000 D
Large molecules removal **Upper limit** (MW)	None	3000 000 D
Vascular access	Peripheral vein, CVC, AVF	CVC, AVF
Blood pump rate (ml/min)	50–150	90–200
Anticoagulation	Citrate, heparin	Heparin, citrate
Procedure time	Shorter	Longer
Adverse events	Platelet loss	Hemolysis, filter failure
Pediatric patients	Older children	Younger children
Device	Specific for cPEX	CRRT compatible

D daltons, *MW* molecular weight, *CVC* central venous catheter, *AVF* arteriovenous fistula, *cPEX* centrifugal plasma exchange, *CRRT* continuous renal replacement therapy

Plasma Removal Efficacy and Clearance of Plasma Proteins

Plasma removal efficacy Plasma removal efficacy (PRE) is defined as the ratio between filtered plasma and total volume of processed plasma per unit of time. It was already mentioned that PRE is higher in cPEX (approx. 80%) and lower in mPEX (30–35%), resulting in longer therapeutic times for mPEX [1]. However, this term defines the removal all plasma proteins and does not give information about the removal of different plasma components after the procedure. Clinically more important is the removal of plasma components during PEX, which is evaluated by measuring their concentrations prior to and after PEX.

Removal of plasma proteins in plasma exchange The clearance of several plasma proteins has been evaluated—immunoglobulins (IgG, IgM, IgA), fibrinogen, immune complexes, and cryoglobulins [17, 22, 23]. Earlier studies also evaluated the effective removal of C3, C4 proteins of the complement system, as well as alpha 1-antitrypsin and alpha 2-macroglobulin [24]. Studies demonstrate similar removal of plasma components in mPEX and cPEX [22].

Plasma protein removal was reported to be 60–70% of the initial concentration of the protein fraction in exchanging 1–1.5 plasma volumes per procedure. Higher plasma volumes do not lead to significant increase in protein removal with PEX, but are associated with longer treatment times and higher risk for complications (clotting of the circuit or filter) [25]. The following parameters for each plasma protein are important in PEX:

- Molecular weight (MW)—the major plasma proteins differ in molecular weight, ranging from 65 kD (albumin), 150 kD [immunoglobulin G(IgG)], 950 kD for immunoglobulin M (IgM), up to 2400 kD for β-lipoprotein [1, 23]. In cPEX, due to the lack of semipermeable membrane, there is no upper MW limit for the clearance of plasma fractions. As already mentioned, current membranes for mPEX provide adequate removal of molecules with MW up to 3,000,000 D. Thus, maximal sieving coefficients for albumin, IgM, and β-lipoprotein (~ 1) are achieved.

- Intravascular distribution—in PEX, only intravascular proteins are removed. However, intravascular proteins are not present in the intravascular space only—e.g., almost 55% of total IgG are detected in the extravascular compartment of the body. Thus, a second protein pool for autoantibodies, cryoglobulins, and immune complexes is present, which is clinically important as these pathological proteins can diffuse from the extravascular space in blood after PEX, thus resulting in rebound of target molecules. Generally, intravascular proportion for IgA, IgG, and IgE ranges between 40 and 45%. Higher intravascular distribution is observed for IgM (78%), IgD (75%), and fibrinogen (80%) [1].
- Rebound of target proteins after PEX—rebound is due to resynthesis of the protein and intravascular transfer from the second pool in extravascular space. Half-life ($T_{1/2}$) for plasma proteins usually ranges between 2 days for C3 protein to 22 days (IgG) [23, 26]. Shorter protein $T_{1/2}$ is associated with faster protein synthesis, compensating for the more rapid catabolism. However, this increases the risk for post-PEX rebound of the target molecules. It should be noted that $T_{1/2}$ for Bence-Jones proteins is increased in poorer kidney function [26]. The transfer from extravascular space of large proteins occurs at the rate of 1–3% per hour. Additionally, fractional turnover of plasma proteins reflects their catabolism rate. IgG molecules have relatively low turnover (7% per day), compared to IgM (19%/day) and 56% (C3) [26].

  Ideally, the target molecule should have high intravascular distribution and long plasma half-life; thus, larger quantity of the molecule will be removed after a single PEX procedure, with minimal risk for post-procedure rebound.

Clinical importance of molecule kinetics in PEX Considering the abovementioned parameters and taking into consideration the nature of the pathological plasma molecule, the most appropriate

PEX treatment can be prescribed, by defining the frequency and number of the procedures.

- IgG molecule—IgG are the predominant type of target molecule in autoimmune diseases. Approximately 45% of IgG are in the intravascular space and have longer half-time (22 days) with low fractional turnover (7% daily). Due to the modest intravascular distribution, a single PEX procedure will not be able to significantly reduce IgG molecules. A rebound due to transfer from extravascular space occurs; the rate of re-synthesis is relatively low. Therefore several PEX procedures (3–6) are needed, with inter-procedure interval 24–48 h to achieve significant reduction of IgG. It has been demonstrated 90% of IgG reduction after 6 PEX procedures with exchange of 1 plasma volume per procedure [26].
- IgM molecule—IgM has high intravascular distribution (80%), with low half-life and more rapid fractional turnover per day (19%). Therefore, it would be effectively removed by a single PEX procedure, but a more rapid re-synthesis may occur, requiring additional PEX. In this case, interval between procedures of 24 and 48 h is suggested. However, in Waldenström disease, 1–3 PEX procedures achieve significant clinical and laboratory effect [27].
- Fibrinogen (Fibr)—the removal of Fibr is a safety issue in PEX, as its plasma removal can cause hemorrhagic event, especially in levels below 1.25 g/l [2]. Its intravascular distribution is approx. 80%; thus, a large fraction of Fibr is removed by a single PEX procedure. Our studies also demonstrate a most significant decrease in fibrinogen after mPEX, compared to other plasma protein fractions evaluated, substituting with albumin solutions only [28]. Due to its relatively short half-life (4.2 days, fractional turnover 25% daily), it has a relatively rapid re-synthesis [26]. However, more than 72 h are needed for Fibr to reach its pre-procedure levels. In order to avoid severe Fibr reduction and increased bleeding risk (e.g., alveolar hemorrhage, 48 h within surgery/biopsy), fresh frozen

plasma can be added to the substitution fluid or infused after PEX.

- Factor VIII—its intravascular distribution is approx. 70%, but its fractional turnover is very high (150% daily) and a shorter half-life of 0.6 days, thus explaining its very quick rebound after PEX and quick return to pre-procedure levels within 4 h after PEX [25].

Mechanism of Action of PEX

As already mentioned, large plasma molecules, especially immunoglobulins have longer half-lives. Therefore, conservative treatment targets the production of new pathological molecules, but the already synthesized ones are still present in patient's circulation, causing damage to target organs. PEX directly removes these molecules and combined with immunosuppressive treatment (in most of the cases) directly improves outcomes in certain clinical scenarios. The use of immunosuppressive agents in PEX will be discussed later.

PEX not only removes pathological proteins, but it was demonstrated to affect cellular immunity too. PEX effectively caused immunomodulation of T cell functions, by shifting the Th_1/Th_2 ratio toward Th_2 cells. PEX reduced the synthesis of Interleukin 2 (IL2) and interferon γ (IFNγ) [29].

Finally, in PEX, vitally important components can be substituted (e.g., correction of ADAMTS 13 enzyme deficiency in thrombotic thrombocytopenic purpura, by substituting with normal FFP, having normal ADAMTS13 activity).

Selective Techniques for Plasmapheresis

Standard PEX separates unselectively plasma from blood cells. Thus, key plasma components (e.g., fibrinogen) are lost during the procedure increasing the risk for adverse events, especially bleeding. In order to improve procedure tolerability, selective techniques for therapeutic plasmapheresis have been developed, reducing the loss of vitally important plasma constituents and requiring less or no substitution. Generally, they are based on membrane plasma separation.

Double Plasmapheresis/Cascade Filtration

In double filtration plasmapheresis (DFPP) or cascade filtration, after the initial separation of plasma from blood cells, additional filtration of plasma occurs by using a second filter with smaller pores (in the range of 0.01–0.03 μm) [2]. The second filtration aims at separating plasma proteins into larger (Ig, immune complexes) and smaller molecules (e.g., albumin). The filtered small proteins are returned to the patient, whereas larger molecules are removed from the body. In this way, lower volumes of replacement fluid are needed. By choosing the second filter (referred as plasma component separator), the removal of specific molecules can be targeted and the volume of substitution fluid can be changed, mainly due to different pore sizes of the plasma component separator. For example, the plasma component separator Cascadeflo EC (Asahi Kasei Medical, Tokyo, Japan) has four different modifications: EC20W, EC30W, EC40W, and EC 50 W. Cascadeflo EC20W filters small protein molecules (albumin), and 20% of processed plasma are discarded; human albumin substitution is required. In contrast, Cascadeflo EC 50 W is designed for LDL particles' removal and larger part of plasma is returned to the patient; no substitution is needed [30].

A major obstacle to wider DFPP use was the inconsistent sieving behavior of the second filter (sieving coefficient for albumin varies between 0.4 and 0.8) [3]. However, with the evolution of devices, the technique will play greater role in clinical practice. Figure 2.6 demonstrates the principles of DFPP.

A modification of DFPP is rheopheresis, in which a rheofilter, filtering lipid molecules, fibrinogen, and IgM is used at the second step of filtration. The method was designed to improve microcirculation and is used for lipoprotein apheresis. The technique will be discussed later in this chapter.

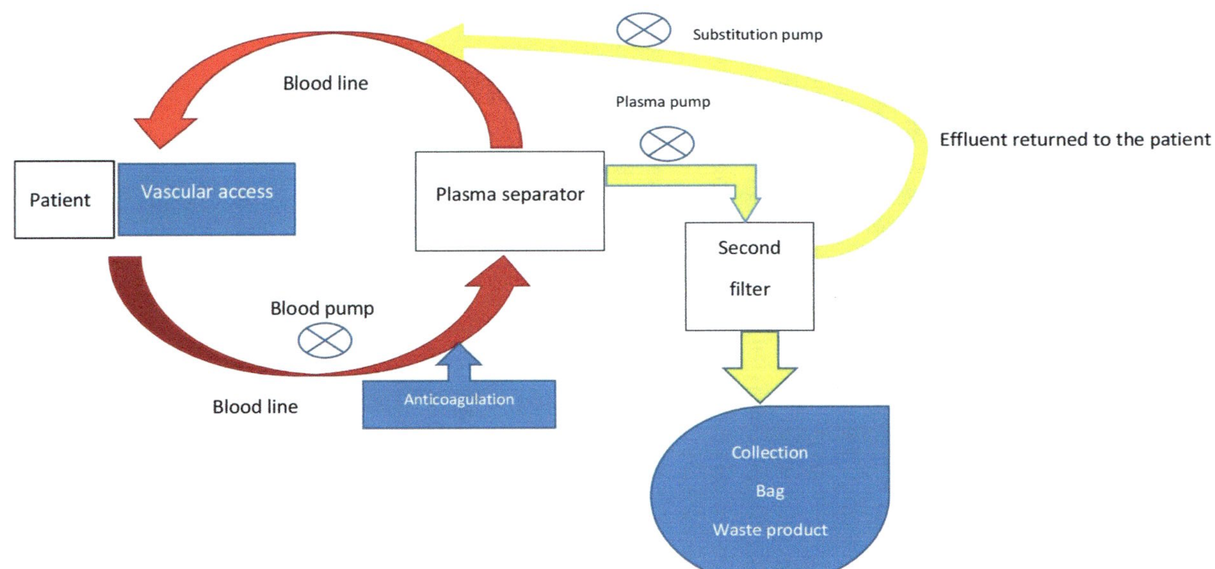

Fig. 2.6 Double filtration plasmapheresis—diagram

Cryofiltration and Thermofiltration

Cryofiltration Cryofiltration is another semiselective technique, aiming at the removal of cryoglobulins. After initial separation, plasma runs through the second filter, where low temperature is applied (+4 °C). In these conditions, cryoglobulins precipitate that are removed as plasma runs through the second filter. Filtered plasma proteins are returned to the patient after heating to normal body temperature.

Thermofiltration This is another type of double filtration plasmapheresis, in which warming up of separated plasma is performed. At temperatures in the range of 38–40 °C, very low density lipoproteins (VLDL) and low density lipoproteins (LDL) form aggregates, which are filtered by the second membrane from high density lipoproteins (HDL). A key disadvantage of thermofiltration is the unknown impact of higher temperatures on other protein fractions [3].

Both cryofiltration and thermofiltration have limited use in practice.

Selective PEX

Selective PEX is based on the use of filter with smaller pores (diameter of 0.03 μm), which is approx. 10 times smaller than standard PEX [e.g., Evacure EC-4A10 (Kawasumi Laboratories Inc., Tokyo, Japan)]. Selective PEX demonstrated poorer removal of IgG, but practically no loss of Fibr, compared to standard PEX [31].

Adsorption

In adsorption, pathological molecules in blood are removed by adhering to sorbents. Sorbents can remove certain molecules selectively or they can adsorb different molecules unselectively.

In adsorption, either the whole blood runs through the adsorber (hemoadsorption), or plasma is initially separated (initial plasmapheresis) and runs through the adsorbent without blood cells (plasma adsorption). Both centrifugal and membrane plasma separation are possible, but centrifugal separation is less preferred, as plasma may contain platelets, which may compromise adsorber function.

Nonselective Adsorption

Hemoadsorption Hemoadsorption is a method, developed mainly for treating exogenous intoxication. In principle, blood is pumped into a filter, containing substance that adsorbs toxic substances (e.g., active charcoal). Hemoadsorption has been used also in the treatment of advanced liver disease. Additionally, it has been tried in oncology, by removing certain aminoacids (L-Tryptophan, L-asparginase), thus blocking tumor growth [3]. Adsorbers for selective hemoadsorption were created too. Polymyxin B–coated adsorbers were used for selective hemoadsorption of endotoxin in the treatment of gram- negative sepsis [32]. Polyvinyl-pyrrolidone–coated adsorbers (CytoSorb®, CytoSorbents Inc., Princeton, NJ, USA) are used in the treatment of crush syndrome and sepsis [33]. Figure 2.7.

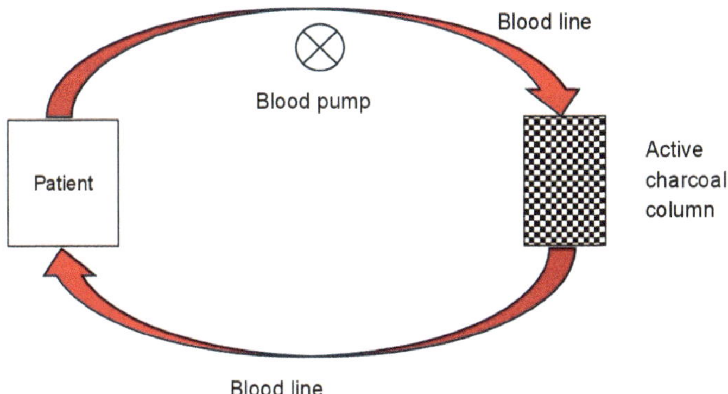

Fig. 2.7 Nonselective hemoadsorption—diagram (active charcoal column)

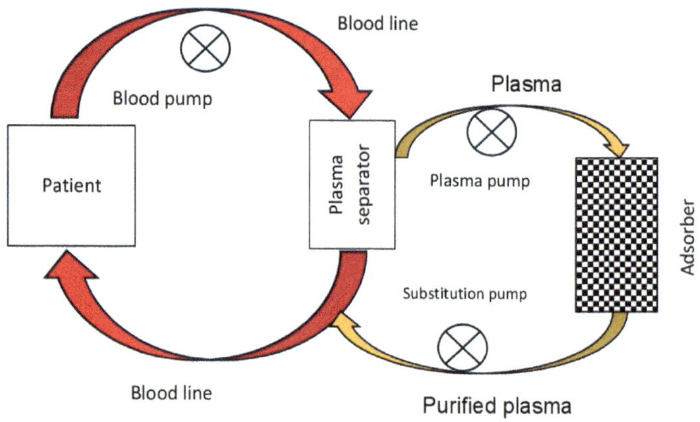

Fig. 2.8 Plasma adsorption—diagram

Plasma adsorption In plasma adsorption, plasma is initially separated from blood cells and is afterward filtered through the charcoal—Fig. 2.8. Similar to hemoadsorption, its main clinical indication is exogenous poisoning. Plasma adsorption is currently the preferred method due to lower complications rate and improved efficacy. Toxin adsorption is improved mainly due to the lower viscosity of plasma, compared to whole blood [3]. Liver failure is another indication for plasma adsorption.

A modification of the technique is effectively used in these cases; a selective adsorbent *styrene divinylbenzene copolymer* is applied for selective removal of bilirubin and bile acids (e.g., PLASORBA ® BR-350(L), Asahi Kasei Medical Co. LTD, Japan).

Selective Adsorption

In selective adsorption, special adsorbers are developed, which remove only certain plasma proteins. Generally, they consist of matrix, in which the specific binding molecule is incorporated. Blood runs through the adsorber and the target plasma molecule is removed from the circulation by reacting with the binding molecule.

However, in most of the cases, plasma is initially separated from blood and undergoes selective adsorption, thus combining plasmapheresis and adsorption. Several selective methods were developed.

Protein-A Immunoadsorption (IA) Protein A is a peptide molecule from the cell wall of *Staphylococcus aureus*. Protein-A-coated adsorbers were found to remove selectively IgG molecules almost 40 years ago, by binding the Fc part of IgG. Protein-A based IA is currently widely used as selective adsorption method. The technique is gaining more popularity, especially in cases were standard PEX has failed to achieve therapeutic results [3]. In addition, practically no substitution fluid is required. The major principles of IA are demonstrated in Fig. 2.9.

Initially plasma is separated from blood. Plasma is transferred to two adsorbent columns, containing Protein-A. Firstly, plasma is filtered through adsorber column 1. After passing through the column, purified plasma is returned to the patient. After 7–20 min, plasma is directed to the second adsorber column, whereas in the meantime, the first one is rinsed with acidic solution and afterward buffering solution. Thus, the adsorbed IgG molecules are removed from protein A in the column and are discarded in the waste bag. Once column 1 is ready for another cycle, plasma is transferred back through it, whereas column 2 is being rinsed and prepared for the next cycle.

Single adsorber regenerative immunoadsorption systems were also developed (Ligasorb ® column, Fresenius Medical CareAG & Co. KGaA, Bad Homburg, Germany, used with the ADAsorb ® device, Medicap Clinic GmbH, Ulrichstein, Germany) [34].

Usually, in IA 2 to 3 plasma volumes are being treated, though theoretically larger treatment volumes can be prescribed. In addition, adequate anticoagulation is required, usually heparin in the blood line and citrate in the plasma line are applied, or citrate only [3, 35].

Synthetic binding proteins Peptide-GAM, used in the adsorbers Globaffin® (Fresenius Medical Care, Germany) was found to be as effective as Protein A adsorbers in the removal of IgG [36].

Alternatively, IA can be performed by using a single adsorption column. However, lower plasma volumes are treated, with shorter treatment times [3]—Fig. 2.10.

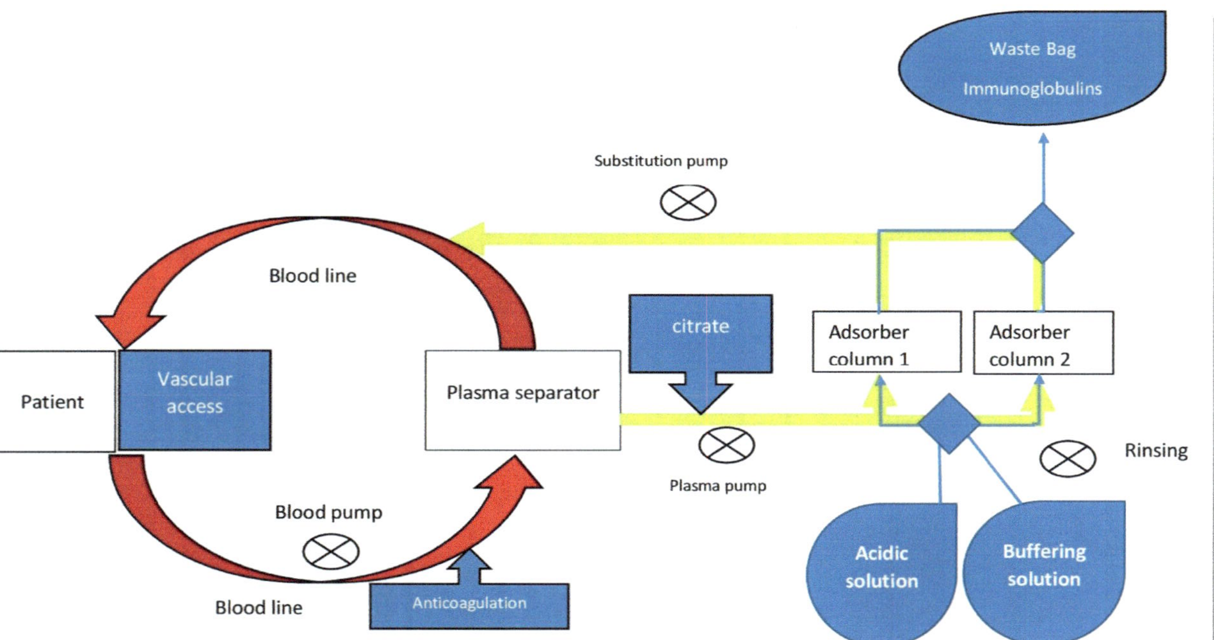

Fig. 2.9 Immunoadsorption—diagram

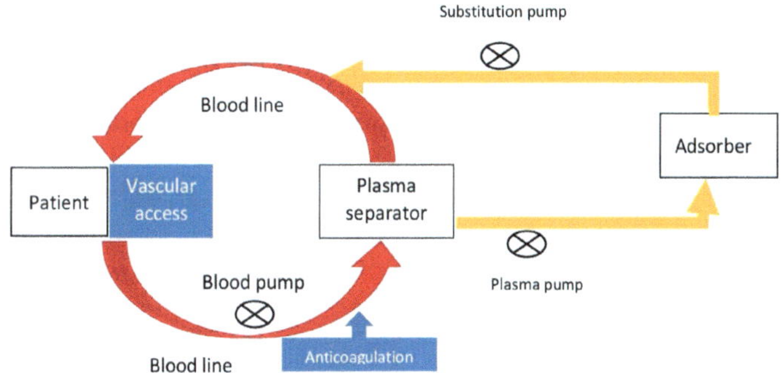

Fig. 2.10 Immunoadsorption—single immunoadsorption column

Other semiselective and selective adsorbers Several other adsorption techniques exist:

- Columns, consisting of polyvinyl alcohol gel matrix coated with tryptophan, demonstrated good effectiveness in eliminating anti-acetylcholine receptor antibodies from plasma, thus influencing the treatment of several neurological diseases, especially in treatment-resistant patients. Initially, plasma is separated from whole blood and runs through the tryptophan-coated adsorber; usually 2.0–2.5 L of plasma are processed per procedure [37].
- Adsorbent, based on polyvinyl alcohol gel, coated with phenylalanine, was used for the treatment of systemic lupus erythematosus (SLE), rheumatoid arthritis, and multiple sclerosis. It was found superior to conservative therapy alone in SLE [38].
- Dextran sulfate–based adsorption was found effective in removing anti-dsDNA antibodies in SLE [39].
- By planting antigens or antibodies in the matrix, selective IA can be performed, as the removal of target molecules is based in antigen-antibody reaction. Example for this type of IA is the removal of LDL, factor VIII inhibitors, soluble tumor necrosis factor–α Receptor type 1 (sTNF R1) [3]. A/B antigen-coated adsorbers are used for removing isoagglutinins in AB0 incompatible transplantation (e.g., Glycosorb® ABO immunoadsorption column) [40].

Unfortunately, the abovementioned adsorbers are rarely used in clinical practice due to the limited range of indications and high cost. What is more, tryptophan-based IA and dextran sulfate columns can cause increased conversion of kininogen to bradykinin. Angiotensin-converting enzyme (ACE) inhibitors block the metabolism of bradykinin, thus increasing its levels, which in turn may cause hypotension. Therefore, ACE inhibitors should not be used in these cases. The topic is discussed in the following sections of this chapter [35].

Lipoprotein Apheresis

Lipoprotein apheresis (LA) is an invasive method for treating dyslipidemia, when life style modifications and conservative treatment have failed to control hypercholesterolemia. Its major indication is homozygous or heterozygous familial hypercholesterolemia (FH) with LDL concentrations above 300 mg/dl (7.76 mmol/L). Heterozygous patients for FH are also indicated for LDL apheresis if they have increased risk for cardiovascular disease (CVD) and LDL >250 mg/dl (5.16 mmol/L) or the presence of CVD or diabetes and LDL > 160 mg/dl (4.14 mmol/L) [41]. Currently its indications span beyond the treatment of hypercholesterolemia, as successful use of LA was reported in focal segmental glomerulosclerosis in children and in adults [42]. The clinical aspects of LA will be discussed in different chapters of this book.

Several options for LDL removal exist.

- Immunoadsorption—LDL removal is based on the antigen-antibody reaction. After initial separation, plasma flows through columns, containing antibodies against apolipoprotein B100 (ApolB100), which is the plasma protein carrier of LDL molecule. LDL/ApolB100 complexes bind to the antibodies, whereas LDL-free plasma is returned to the patient. Generally, the process resembles protein-A IA, depicted in Fig. 2.9. Once column 1 is saturated, plasma flow is redirected to column 2. In the meantime, column 1 is regenerated by using acidic solution, which breaks the covalent bond between LDL/ApolB100 and anti-ApolB100 antibodies; LDL/ApolB100 molecules are washed away and the binding potential of the antibodies on the column is restored. LDL IA requires 3–6 L of plasma volume for each treatment, achieving up to 40% reduction from pre-treatment LDL levels [3]. The procedure is relatively safe, but has a high cost. Additionally, the use of ACE inhibitors in this type of LA is contraindicated, due to the risk for bradykinin accumulation [43].

- Heparin–induced extracorporeal LDL precipitation (HELP)—This type of lipoprotein apheresis is based on the principle of DFPP; LDL molecules are removed by precipitation after being treated with acidic solution of heparin. Initially, plasma is separated from blood; at the second stage, plasma is being processed with acidic solution of heparin; at the third stage, plasma runs through a second filter, removing LDL-heparin precipitates; at the fourth stage, heparin is removed by heparin adsorber. Finally, plasma undergoes bicarbonate dialysis, restoring physiological pH and is returned to the patient. The procedure achieves up to 50% reduction of pre-treatment LDL levels. However, heparin forms precipitates with plasma proteins, most importantly fibrinogen. As a significant fibrinogen depletion is present, treatment volume is limited to 3 l [3]. In HELP, the use of ACE inhibitors is not contraindicated [43].
- Double filtration lipid apheresis—the method is again based on DFPP, with a second filter used for removal of lipoproteins, LDL molecules, and triglycerides. Usually rheofilters are used, which improve microcirculation by effectively removing LDL, VLDL, triglyceride molecules, but also fibrinogen and IgM (e.g., Rheofilter ER-4000 ®, Asahi Kasei Medical Co. LTD, Japan). The method achieved similar effectiveness (70% LDL reduction) to the HELP technique, requiring plasma volume of 2500–3500 ml [44]. Yet, it is far more simplified, compared to HELP. High permeability plasma component separators are used for LA too, as they selectively remove LDL molecules (e.g., Cascadeflo EC50W, Asahi Kasei Medical, Tokyo, Japan; FRACTIOsmart™ Large, Medica S.p.A., Medolla, Italia). In addition, a recent study demonstrated that polyethersulfone had better biocompatibility to ethylene-vinyl alcohol copolymer in double filtration lipid apheresis [45]. Rheopheresis demonstrated promising results in the treatment of peripheral

artery disease, calciphylaxis, and age-related macular degeneration [46].

- Dextran sulfate–based lipoprotein apheresis—the process resembles IA, depicted in Fig. 2.10. After initial separation from blood cells, plasma flows through columns, consisting of cellulose-dextran sulfate. Dextran sulfate is negatively charged and binds to positively charged ApolB100, carrying LDL molecules. After saturation of the column, rinsing and regeneration are performed. The procedure achieves up to 80% LDL reduction, but a drop in fibrinogen and factor VIII is also present. ACE inhibitors can also cause hypotension by increasing bradykinin levels during dextran sulfate–based LDL apheresis [41]. The use of regenerative columns enables the use of higher treatment plasma volumes (up to 6 liters).
- Direct adsorption of lipoproteins (DALI) is based on the principles of hemoperfusion (Fig. 2.7). Blood runs directly through an adsorber, covered with negatively charged polyacrylate molecules. They bind to the positively charged apolipoproteins, thus removing LDL and VLDL. Usually 1.5–2 blood volumes are being, resulting in LDL reduction by 60%. A recent study however demonstrated that DALI method is inferior to double filtration lipid apheresis [47]. Additionally, ACE inhibitors can cause bradykinin accumulation in DALI.

Plasmapheresis, Combined with Other Replacement/Elimination Methods

Tandem PEX/Hemodialysis (TPEX/HD)

A certain subtype of patients may need dialysis and PEX. Performed separately, several hours may be required for these two procedures. Therefore, tandem techniques, combining PEX and dialysis were developed, providing optimal removal of toxins and pathological macromolecules simultaneously for a shorter period of time. Generally, both cPEX and mPEX can be used in TPEX/HD [48]. The method was effectively used in the treatment of ANCA vasculitis, AB0 desensitization, and even plasma cell disorders. Practically, the blood is pumped out of the patient; the PEX circuit branches after blood is drawn from the patient; two parallel circuits (dialysis and plasma exchange) are formed; plasma containing pathological Ig is discarded and a substitution fluid is infused back into blood; afterward the whole blood joins the dialysis circuit, undergoes dialysis, and is returned to the patient—Fig. 2.11 [49].

Alternatively, the dialyzer can be placed prior to plasma separator; first, the whole blood is dialyzed, then plasma separation is performed, as plasma circuit branches the dialysis one. After substitution fluid is added to blood cells concentrate, the whole blood is returned to the patient [50]—Fig. 2.11b.

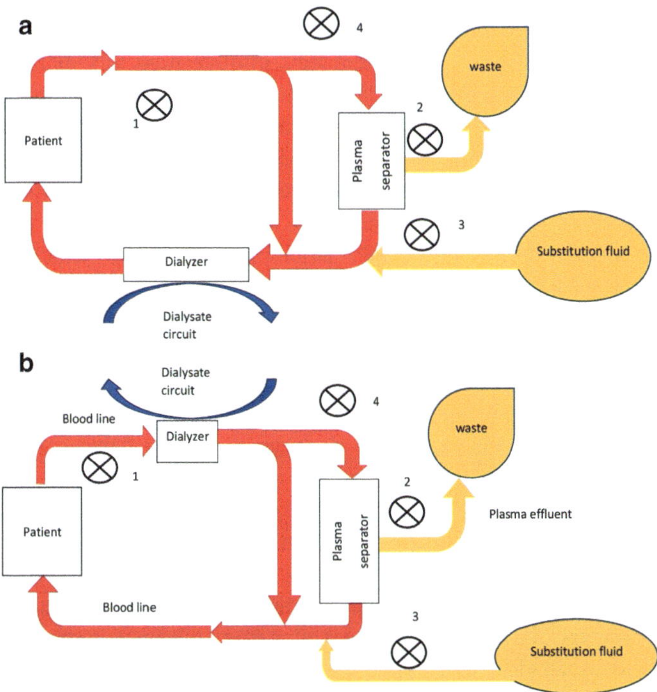

Fig. 2.11 (**a**) Tandem PEX/HD, dialyzer placed after plasma separator—diagram. (**b**) Tandem PEX/HD, dialyzer prior to plasma separator—diagram

Liver Supporting Systems

In liver failure, the major goal is removal of water-insoluble toxins (bilirubin, bile acids). It cannot be achieved by current dialysis methods. Several methods have been developed so far [51]: PEX, the molecular adsorbent recirculating system (MARS®, Gambro, Sweden), single pass albumin dialysis (SPAD), and the Fractionated Plasma Separation and Adsorption System (FPSA; Prometheus ®, Fresenius, Germany).

- PEX—in liver failure, high volumes of plasma are removed and are substituted with fresh frozen plasma. The method demonstrated effectiveness in treatment of hepatic encephalopathy, but the need for large volume of fresh plasma for substitution is a disadvantage of the method [52].
- SPAD—blood of the patient runs through high flux dialyzer diffusion limited to 30 kDa. The dialysate contains 1–3% albumin. Hydrophobic toxins, that accumulate in liver failure, cross the membrane by diffusion, bind to the free binding sites of albumin dialysate and are washed away. The method reduces levels of urea and creatinine too.
- MARS—blood flows into albumin-coated filter, which is impermeable to albumin; a counter current albumin containing circuit is formed, which carries away albumin-bound toxins from the membrane by binding them to the free binding sites of the countercurrent albumin solution; afterward, albumin is detoxicated by two adsorption columns (removing hydrophobic toxins) and additional dialyzer, removing water-soluble toxins and finally is recirculated in the filter, binding to new toxins (recirculation of exogenous albumin).
- Fractionated Plasma Separation and Adsorption System (FPSA; Prometheus ®, Fresenius, Germany) is based on fractionated separation of albumin. Patient's blood runs through a special plasma separator (Albuflow® membrane), permeable to molecules with upper molecular weight up to 250 kDa. Practically the membrane is permeable to albumin and albumin-bound toxins. The separated albumin is detoxified by using two adsorption columns (removing hydrophobic toxins)

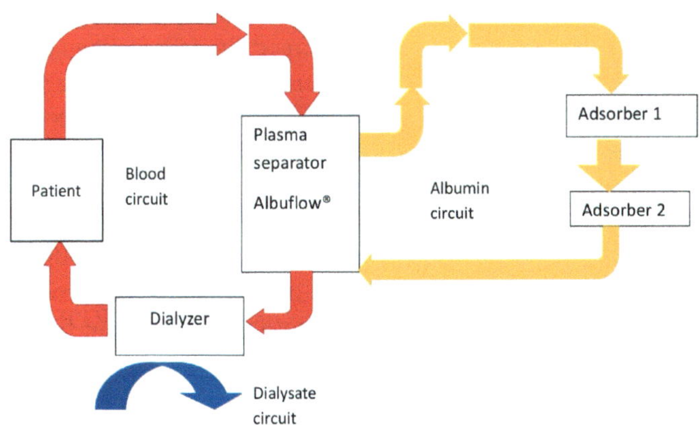

Fig. 2.12 Fractionated Plasma Separation and Adsorption System (FPSA; Prometheus ®, Fresenius, Germany) liver support system—diagram

and is returned to blood circulation. The blood undergoes further detoxication (high flux dialysis, removing water-soluble toxins) and is returned to the patient (Fig. 2.12).

Vascular Access in Plasma Exchange

Vascular access (VA) for PEX is vitally important for the success of the procedure. Inadequate access causes poor blood flow throughout the circuit, may cause frequent stops of the blood flow due to inadequate pressures along the system, which in turn increases the risk for clotting of the circuit or plasma separator, thus finally leading to early ending and failure of PEX. Therefore, a careful evaluation of each patient is needed and all vascular options should be taken into consideration.

Several types of access in PEX exist, according to the type of vessel used:

1. Peripheral VA – using peripheral veins. Mostly used in cPEX, due to the lower blood rates of the method. Peripheral vein cannulation is generally preferred to central vein use due to its better safety profile. Several requirements are present for peripheral

VA: stable patient, adequate peripheral vein anatomy, short PEX treatment – up to 10 days, cPEX modality [53]. It should be mentioned that in lipid apheresis peripheral VA can be used successfully too[47]. Generally, metal venous cannula, size 16 - 19 Gauge is used for the inlet line. Larger arm veins are used - e.g. cephalic/basilic/antecubital veins. Ultrasound guided technique for placing the inlet cannula have widely been introduced in clinical practice, reducing complications rate during needling. The widely used Intravenous non-metal cannulas are avoided for inlet option as they may collapse during drawing blood. However, they can be effectively used in outlet lines, smaller veins for the return line can be used too [54].

Additional devices for peripheral VA were evaluated:

- Hard non-metal IV cannulas—these devices were developed for needling arteriovenous fistulas (AVFs) mainly. They consist of specific plastic material, which does not collapse during blood drawing and usually have side holes along the catheter (e.g., Supercath™, model NEO, PRO and Clampcath, Medikit Co. Ltd., Tokyo, Japan). Current guidelines recommend their use in AVFs needling together with metal venous cannulas, though studies do not demonstrate superiority of non-metal venous catheters to metal ones in terms of safety or reduced pain [55]. In addition, larger and harder intravenous cannulas were associated with higher rate of phlebitis of peripheral veins [56].
- Midlines—these catheters are longer peripheral VA devices, used when longer conservative treatment is needed. Their insertion is based on the Seldinger method, usually veins proximal to cubital fossa are needled. The tip of the midlines lies in the axilla level; midlines can be single- or double-lumen devices. They achieve flows up to 80 ml/min, with diameters 16–18 Gauge; however, their length is an obstacle for wider use.

2. Peripherally inserted central catheters (PICC)—these catheters are central lines, which are inserted in peripheral vein and their tip reaches the lower segment of superior vena cava or

right atrium. PICC have failed to achieve adequate blood flows in PEX, and their use is not recommended in PEX [53].

3. Central venous catheter (CVC), dialysis compatible, are usually divided into two subtypes—non-tunneled and tunneled CVC and are used both for mPEX and cPEX. The tip should be located in the lower segment of superior vena cava or right atrium in order to provide adequate blood flows. Ultrasound-guided placement of CVC is generally recommended.
   - Non-tunneled CVC—the catheters are temporary ones and are used for short-term PEX. The major insertion sites are subclavian veins and internal jugular veins; femoral vein cannulation is avoided due to the increased risk for infection and deep vein thrombosis. The advantages of non-tunneled CVC are immediate use after insertion and easy removal after PEX is ended. The disadvantages are mainly associated with the insertion of the CVC—the need for qualified personnel, risks for infection, deep vein thrombosis, central vein stenosis, pneumothorax, etc. Non-tunneled CVC are used in short-term PEX (duration within 10 days).
   - Tunneled CVC (tCVC)—inserted after cannulation of internal jugular vein is performed. This type of VA is used in mid- and long-term PEX, lasting more than 10 days [53]. Tunneled CVC share similar advantages and disadvantages with non-tunneled CVC; however, expertise is needed in removing these catheters.
4. Arteriovenous fistula (AVF) and arteriovenous graft (AVG)—these VA are widely used in dialysis patients. In PEX, they are in cases where chronic PEX is performed (more than 1 year). Needling of AVF can be performed by metal and non-metal catheters; AVGs should be needled with metal catheters only. This type of VA has the advantage of longer use, providing adequate blood flow rates. The disadvantages are also significant—risk for steal syndrome, thrombosis, and need for qualified personnel to needle the VA. Generally, AVF have lower rates for thrombosis and infection, compared to AVGs. It was demonstrated that AVF/AVG had poorer patency and maturation rates in non-dialysis patient vs. patients on hemodialysis

[57]. The results probably reflect the influence of chronic inflammatory disease on AVF/AVG maturation.

5. Venous ports (VP)—Venous ports (VP) consist of tunneled CVC in the internal jugular vein, attached to a special chamber, which is implanted subcutaneously. Thus, the catheter is fully implanted beneath the skin, which reduces the risk for infections and accidental removal. Venous ports are used for long-term PEX, both mPEX and cPEX [53]. VP apheresis is associated with higher incidence of clotting of the circuit. Other complications with VP are membrane degradation, extravasation, and infection. For adequate PEX, two single-lumen VP can be implanted or single VP for inlet line and peripheral cannula for return line [1]; double-lumen ports were also developed.

Two types of VP are present [54]:

- Standard VP—the catheters can be used successfully in cases where low blood flow is needed (60–100 ml/min).
- Apheresis VP—specialized VP for PEX were developed, suitable for all types PEX procedures [e.g., Titan-Port APH (PakuMed® medical products GMBH, Essen, Germany); PowerFlow® (BD)]. Their use in PEX has demonstrated significant improvement in cost- and time-effectiveness, compared to standard VP [58].

According to the needling technique, two options are present—single needle (SN) method and double needle (DN) method. In SN PEX, one needle is used for drawing blood and blood return. The method was used in mPEX almost 40 years ago. Currently, the use of SN-PEX is limited to cPEX. In DN-PEX, inlet and outlet sites are different and the technique is preferred in mPEX, as higher blood flows are needed; additionally, discontinuous flow would increase the risk for filter clotting. A recent study compared SN-cPEX to DN-cPEX. SN-cPEX demonstrated similar plasma removal efficacy and safety profile with better tolerability of the patients to DN-cPEX, despite longer treatment times [59]. Table 2.2 summarizes the characteristics of vascular access options in PEX.

Table 2.2 Vascular access characteristics in plasma exchange [53, 54, 57]

Type of VA	Type of device	PEX type	PEX duration	Advantages	Disadvantages
Peripheral vein	Metal catheter (i/o)	cPEX	Short	Less complications	Low BFR Thrombophlebitis
	Non-metal catheters (i/o)	cPEX	Short and long term	Less complications	Low BFR Higher thrombophlebitis rate
	Standard IV cannulas—Outlet only	cPEX	Short and long term	Less complications	Low BFR Thrombophlebitis
	Midlines	cPEX	Short and long term	Less complications	Low flow rate
CVC	Non-tunneled	cPEX/mPEX	Short (less than 10 days)	Immediate use, easy removal High BFR	Infections, stenosis, thrombosis, pneumothorax
	Tunneled	cPEX/mPEX	More than 10 days, incl. Very long duration	Immediate use High BFR	Infections, stenosis, thrombosis, pneumothorax
Peripherally inserted central catheters	Not recommended in PEX				

(continued)

Table 2.2 (continued)

Type of VA	Type of device	PEX type	PEX duration	Advantages	Disadvantages
AVF/AVG	Metal catheters (i/o) The only option for AVG	cPEX/mPEX	More than 1 year	Good BFR Less infections	Steal syndrome, thrombosis Need for qualified personnel
	Non-metal catheters (i/o)	cPEX/mPEX	More than 1 year	Good BFR Less infections	Steal syndrome, thrombosis Need for qualified personnel
Venous ports	Standard VP	cPEX/mPEX	More than 1 year	Fully implanted	Membrane degradation, clotting, infection, extravasation
	Apheresis VP	cPEX/mPEX	More than 1 year	Fully implanted Higher BFR than standard VP	Membrane degradation, clotting, infection, extravasation

PEX plasma exchange, *cPEX* centrifugal plasma exchange, *mPEX* membrane plasma exchange, *BFR* blood flow rate, *CVC* central venous catheter, *AVF* arteriovenous fistula, *AVG* arteriovenous graft, *VP* venous port, *i* inlet line, *o* outlet line

Anticoagulation

Anticoagulation is crucial for the success of PEX by preventing clotting of the circuit. Concomitant diseases (liver disease, renal disease) and medications, as well type of PEX influence anticoagulant choice and dosing.

Circuit Anticoagulation

Two basic options for anticoagulation are present—citrate and heparin.

- Citrate—its anticoagulant effect is due to binding to calcium ions in plasma, thus blocking their physiological function in hemostasis. Citrate preparations [e.g., Anticoagulant Citrate Dextrose solution A or B (ACD-A/ACD-B)] are recommended in PEX techniques with low blood flow rate, as during the circulation in the circuit it is partially cleared (up to 80% in cPEX), without causing systemic effects. Higher blood flow rates can increase citrate load in patient's circulation. Generally, it is the preferred anticoagulant as it has better safety profile and shorter half-time (18–54 min). Citrate has hepatic metabolism, yet up to 35% of it are excreted via the kidneys [60]. Citrate should be used at lowest doses to avoid side effects. Suggested doses are in range of 1.0–1.8 mg/kg/min [61]. Citrate dosing can be prescribed as whole blood: anticoagulant ratio, which should range from 10:1 to 14:1. Finally, individualized approach in dosing citrate has been suggested, based on ionized calcium (iCa) concentrations. Testing for iCa van be performed pre- and post-filter; target concentrations suggested were 0.24–0.33 mmol/L (prefilter) or 0.30–0.40 mmol/l (post-filter in continuous renal replacement therapy) [62, 63]. It should be mentioned that blood products contain citrate as anticoagulant, thus further increasing citrate load (e.g., FFP as substitution fluid in PEX). In these cases, lower citrate dose should be applied. Albumin solutions can bind calcium ions, thus potentiating citrate-associated hypocalcemia, which is the major side effect. Its treatment depends on its presentation: milder forms can be treated with 2 grams calcium carbonate orally, whereas severe forms need intravenous treatment. It has been demonstrated that continuous calcium supplementation in substitution fluid (calcium gluconate, 10 ml/L of 4–5% albumin substitution fluid) prevents hypocalcemia episodes most effectively, compared to oral calcium or calcium gluconate bolus dose [64]. Additional adverse effects are metabolic alkalosis and hypomagnesemia (the latter rarely needs correction; however prophylactic use of magnesium sulfate 3 g every 6 h—total 4 doses was suggested [61]).

- Unfractionated heparin (UFH) is used mainly in mPEX. Heparin exerts its anticoagulant action by binding to antithrombin (AT). The UFH-AT complex inactivates clotting factors, namely, thrombin and factor Xa. Initially, UFH is applied as bolus dose of 2000 to 5000 IU, which is followed by heparin infusion at the rate of 500–2000 IU per hour [2]. The most common adverse event is bleeding; other important complications of heparin use are heparin-induced thrombocytopenia (HIT) and osteoporosis.
- Low molecular heparins (LMH), Naproparin, Enoxaparin, Dalteparin, etc. Their anticoagulant effect is based on binding to AT and inhibiting predominantly factor Xa activity. LMHs have longer half-life than UFH and similar side effects. In our institution, LWHs are given at dose of 0.01 ml/kg as bolus at the beginning of PEX; usually the dose is in the range of 0.8–1.0 ml per procedure.
- Combined UFH and citrate anticoagulation—usually performed when reduction of citrate load is needed. Heparin is either infused simultaneously with citrate infusion or is added to citrate bag (e.g., 5000 IU Heparin are added to 500 ml ACD-A); citrate infusion/dose in these cases is reduced more than twice to achieve safe anticoagulation [61].
- Saline (200–400 ml/h), added to heparin, demonstrated reduction in circuit clotting and can be used in PEX in patients, which have preserved urine output [16].

Concomitant Anticoagulation and PEX

The presence of anticoagulant therapy can increase bleeding risk in PEX. As different strategies have been used, the basic principle is to evaluate and follow up each patient individually.

- UFH—unfractionated heparin can be applied intravenously or subcutaneously. Activated partial thromboplastin time (aPTT) and anti-factor Xa activity are the tests to evaluate its effectiveness. Its half-life is less than 3 h. There are conflicting reports on the management of UFH in PEX patients. According to some authors, heparin infusion should be stopped 1–2 h prior to PEX procedure; however, Kaplan et al. demonstrated a need to increase heparin infusion during PEX in order to keep pre-procedure anti-Xa activity [60, 65]. Reduction in citrate infusion is also recommended.
- LMH—due to their longer half-life, low molecular heparins should be stopped 24 h prior to the procedure. Anti-Xa activity is used to evaluate their action.
- Direct oral anticoagulant (DOAC)—widely used for the treatment of acute thromboembolism and stroke prevention. Generally, anti-Xa activity is used to measure their action (Apixaban, Edoxaban, Rivaroxaban), calibrated for each agent; diluted thrombin time is used for Dabigatran. The assays are not widely available. There is no sufficient data on the use of DOACs in PEX. In cases of bleeding, specific antidotes can be used or plasma infusion. Stopping the DOAC treatment prior to PEX should be considered carefully, taking into consideration the indication for use in every patient [60]. Switching to LMH/UFH is also an option.
- Fondaparinux—used in pulmonary embolism and deep vein thrombosis, its effect is evaluated by Fondaparinux-calibrated anti-Xa activity. Due to its half-life of 13–21 h, treatment

should be stopped 24 h prior to PEX. If anticoagulation is needed, UFH can be used instead.

- Direct thrombin inhibitors (Argatroban, Desirudin)—should be discontinued in high risk patients [60].
- Warfarin—widely used anticoagulant, whose therapeutic effectiveness is evaluated by international normalized ratio (INR) measurement. High INR is a risk for bleeding and vitamin K is used as antidote. Alternatively, fresh frozen plasma can be used. A switching to UFH/LWH prior to PEX is a reasonable approach.
- Aspirin–Platelet function tests are used to evaluate Aspirin effect. If Aspirin-associated bleeding is present, the medication should be stopped and platelet infusions should be considered prior to PEX, though the benefit is uncertain [66].
- Oral platelet inhibitors (thyenopyridines) block P2Y12 receptor on the platelet membrane thus blocking platelet aggregation. Similarly to Aspirin, their effect is measured by platelet function tests. Their use is associated with increased bleeding risk in patients on dialysis or PEX [60]. Unfortunately, platelet infusions failed to demonstrate superiority to standard of care for patients on antiplatelet therapy and hemorrhage.

Substitution Fluids

As plasma during PEX is removed, an adequate substitute fluid is required. The substitution fluid should be equal to the volume of plasma removed and should have similar biological and physiological characteristics (colloid oncotic pressure, coagulation factors, electrolyte composition). Saline products should not be used for substitution, as they cannot keep the physiological osmotic pressure. Generally, protein-containing fluids are used:

- Human albumin solution—human albumin is diluted in isotonic saline. Albumin concentrations varying between 3% and 6% have been used; in our institution, we use 4% human albumin for PEX. The solution is well tolerated. Its major disadvantage is the loss of coagulation factors (especially fibrinogen). It was already mentioned that it takes more than 72 h for Fibr to reach its initial pre-PEX levels. Therefore, several PEX procedures will decrease Fibr levels significantly and may increase bleeding risk. However, in certain situations, such as Fibrinogen <1.25 g/L, prothrombin time increased more than 3 s above normal values, or concomitant coagulopathy (liver failure), FFP should be added to substitution or applied after PEX [2].

- Fresh Frozen Plasma—FFP can be used for substitution fluid, as it fulfills all requirements for substation fluid. However, FFP carries the risk for blood-borne infections (hepatitis, HIV, cytomegalovirus). It is associated with higher risk for anaphylactic reaction than human albumin [67]; it also increases citrate load due to citrate use in blood products. Another disadvantage is the need for large number of donors to provide the needed quantity of FFP for the PEX treatment. Total FFP substitution is indicated in certain cases—most importantly in the treatment of thrombotic thrombocytopenic purpura (TTP) due to severely decreased ADAMTS13 (a disintegrin and metalloproteinase with a thrombospondin type 1 motif, member 13) activity. Total or partial FFP substitution can be performed also in patients with active hemorrhage or high bleeding risk (pulmonary hemorrhage, within 48 h prior to/after biopsy and surgery).
- Cryo-precipitate poor plasma (CPP)—this is plasma in which cryo-precipitates have been removed, resulting in lower concentrations of certain clotting factors (factor VIII, von Wilebrand factor). It has the same indications for substitution in PEX as FFP. A recent meta-analysis demonstrated that CCP is at least not inferior to FFP as substitution in PEX in TTP patient; in the whole pool of patients included, CCP substitution had lower mortality to FFP. Thus, CCP may be a reasonable alternative to FFP in the future [68].
- Gelatine-based solutions—due to their shorter half-lives, compared to albumin, they are not used as substitution in PEX. Additionally, they increase the risk for kidney injury in patients with renal disease.

PEX Prescription

Prescribing the volume of exchanged plasma in PEX is based on the calculation of estimated plasma volume (EPV), using the following simplified equation, suggested by AA Kaplan—Eq. 2.8 [69]:

$$EPV = (0.065 * kg\, BW) * (1 - Hct) \tag{2.8}$$

Treatment volumes in PEX usually vary between 1*EPV and 1.5*EPV. Larger volumes are not required in immune diseases, as they will not significantly improve immunoglobulin removal. However, in metabolic diseases (e.g., fulminant Wilson disease, acute liver failure) higher PEX volumes are used (treatment volume > 1.5 EPV); this type of PEX is also referred as high-volume PEX (HV-PEX).

As already mentioned, in IA larger volumes (2*EPV up to 3*EPV) can be processed [3].

Additionally, adequate substitution and anticoagulation should be administered (see previous chapters).

As already mentioned in section "Plasma removal efficacy and clearance of plasma proteins", frequency and number of needed PEX procedures depends on the target molecule; additionally treatment frequency depends on the type of disease, clinical manifestations in each patient. The type of disease and its presentation may influence also the choice of vascular access (peripheral veins in stable vs. CVC in unstable cases), substitution fluid (human albumin vs. FFP), thus making PEX prescription individual and specific for every patient.

The effectiveness of PEX in different diseases will be discussed later in this chapter and in other chapters of this book.

Medications in Plasma Exchange

Immunosuppression and Biological Agents

PEX removes the present antibodies/antigens in plasma, but the active immune cells are not influenced by the procedure, and the formation of new target molecules (immunoglobulins, immune complexes) continues. Therefore, additional immunosuppression is needed for PEX to have full effect on immune disease. Different immunosuppressive regimens have been suggested in the past. Steroids (CS, 1 mg/kg daily) and cyclophosphamide (CYC, 2–3 mg/kg daily or intravenous boluses) were initially given. Current guidelines recommend use of steroids in combination with cyclophosphamide [70]. Novel agents were also introduced in practice—Rituximab (RTX, 375 mg/m^2/weekly for 4 weeks) and intravenous immunoglobulins (IVIG, e.g., 100 mg/kg after each PEX). Doses and prescription schedule of the medications may vary across different diseases. Another novel agents used in combination with PEX are caplacizumab (in combination with CS and RTX for immune-mediated thrombotic thrombocytopenic purpura) and bortezomib [71, 72]. Immunosuppressive protocols, associated with PEX, vary between different diseases and will be discussed in designated chapters of this book.

Other Medications in PEX

Correction of hypocalcemia and hypomagnesemia has been discussed in previous sections. Additionally, due to lower potassium levels in human albumin, hypokalemia may develop, which may necessitate correction.

Angiotensin-Converting Enzyme (ACE) Inhibitors in PEX

The use of ACE inhibitors requires special attention during PEX, as it may be associated with bradikinin release during the procedure, presenting with hypotension and flushing. Plasma prekalikrein-kinin system may be activated by contacting negatively charged surfaces (membranes, adsorbers). Thus, large amounts of bradykinin are formed by breakdown of kininogen. Physiologically angiotensin-converting enzyme inactivates bradykinin. However, the use of ACE inhibitors blocks bradykinin inactivation, thus causing bradykinin accumulation, leading to anaphylactoid symptoms (e.g., hypotension, flushing).

- Procedures at higher risk: membrane PEX, certain types of membranes and adsorbers are associated with higher risk (e.g., synthetic AN69 polyacrylonitrile membrane, dextrane/tryptophane-based/phenylalanine-based adsorbers), albumin supplementation.
- Avoid use of ACE inhibitors 24–48 h prior to PEX/LA procedure; follow instructions from filter/adsorber's manufacturer; angiotensin receptor blockers (ARB) theoretically may have benefit, but bradykinin-associated symptoms have been described in ARB use too.

Adverse Events, Associated with PEX; Contraindications to PEX

Generally, PEX is well tolerated, if experienced personnel performs the procedure. PEX can be performed even in unstable patients, but in these cases, it should be performed preferably in intensive care units (ICUs). Table 2.3 summarizes the adverse events, associated with plasma exchange.

Table 2.3 Adverse events, associated with plasma exchange [3, 53, 54, 57, 60, 61]

Mechanism	Complications	Prevention
Vascular access—Associated: CVC Peripheral cannulas (PC) Venous ports AVF/AVG	Hematoma (CVC, AVF/AVG) Infection/sepsis (all types of VA) Pneumothorax (CVC) Phlebitis (PC) Thrombosis (CVC) Stenosis (CVC, AVF) Steal syndrome(AVF/AVG) Aneurisms (AVF) Accidental removal (CVC) Inadequate BFR (all types of VA) Need for qualified staff (CVC, AVF/AVG) Port membrane degradation (VP)	Peripheral VA preferred US-guided cannulation Avoid long dwell times In long treatment: Use tCVC/VP/AVF/AVG Experienced staff needed for tCVC/AVF/AVG Adequate post-PEX care
Substitution fluid associated	Anaphylaxis to FFP Death, due to anaphylaxis Coagulopathy and bleeding (HA substitution) Blood-borne infections Citrate overload Hypokalemia	Vital signs monitoring Avoid FFP if previous reactions reported FFP substitution/post-PEX administration if Fibr $^{<}$1.25 g/l Prothrombin time 3 s above normal Consider FFP as substitution fluid in high bleeding risk† or active hemorrhage Reduce citrate dose if FFP needed

(continued)

Table 2.3 (continued)

Mechanism	Complications	Prevention
Anticoagulation-associated	Bleeding Circuit/filter clotting Hypocalcemia Hypomagnesemia Metabolic alkalosis HIT	Vital signs monitoring TMP monitoring iCa monitoring Consider lower citrate/heparin doses Ca/Mg supplementation (oral/intravenous) Stop heparin in HIT
Other Membrane intolerability Bradykinin release (ACE inh in specific membranes/adsorptive columns) High BFR Miscellaneous	Hypotension Dyspnea Low platelet count Hemolysis Drug and vitamin removal Cardiac arrest Pulmonary edema Pulmonary embolism Anaphylactoid reaction Flushing	Consider membrane change if possible Consider different apheresis technique Correct BFR Vital signs and laboratory monitoring Stop ACE inh 24–48 h prior to procedure

CVC central venous catheter, *tCVC* tunneled central venous catheter, *AVF* arterio-venous fistula, *AVG* arterio-venous graft, *VA* vascular access, *PC* peripheral cannula, *VP* venous port, *FFP* fresh frozen plasma, *HA* human albumin, *iCa* ionized calcium, *Ca* calcium, *Mg* magnesium, *Fibr* fibrinogen, *HIT* heparin induced thrombocytopenia, *TMP* transmembrane pressure, *ACE inh* angiotensin-converting enzyme inhibitor, *BFR* blood flow rate, *LDL* low density lipoprotein, † high bleeding risk—patients within 48 h from surgery/biopsy

Other Apheresis Techniques: Cytapheresis

In this section, cytapheresis will be briefly presented. Generally, blood cells are being separated from plasma via centrifugation. The method is used in blood donation [red blood cells (RBCs), platelets (PLT)], as well as treatment in certain diseases (hereditary hemochromatosis, hyperleukocytosis, and inflammatory bowel disease). Cytapheresis for donation will be not be discussed in this book. Three basic modifications are present—erythrocytapheresis (RBC removal), leukocytapheresis (removal of white blood cells), and thrombocytapheresis (PLT removal).

Erythrocytapheresis

Erythrocytapheresis is the selective removal of red blood cells (RBC) from whole blood. The separation is achieved by centrifugation. Removed RBC are substituted with saline or colloids. Erythrocytapheresis is most commonly used for hematocrit reduction in polycytemia vera and hereditary hemochromatosis.

If the procedure is coupled with donor RBC substitution, the procedure is called RBC exchange [mostly used in the treatment of sickle cell disease (SCD)]. In RBC exchange, the pathological erythrocytes and hemoglobins are substituted for normal RBC, thus reducing the risk for iron overload, hematocrit increase, or edema. RBC exchange was found particularly effective in the treatment of acute SCD with stroke [73].

Both types of erythrocytapheresis are performed automatically; however, a manual version of these two treatments is also possible by performing simple phlebotomy. Automatic RBC exchange was found to be superior to manual RBC exchange in terms of control of HbS, lower risk for iron accumulation, and shorter procedure duration. Similarly, automated erythrocytapheresis was found to reduce iron load in hereditary hemochromatosis, compared to phlebotomy [73].

Peripheral cannulas are generally sufficient. Similarly to PEX, in RBC exchange treatment volumes are being calculated.

Practically, 1.5 RBC volumes per procedure are recommended. The following Eqs. 2.9 and 2.10 can be used in calculating the parameters:

$$RBC\,volume = TBV * hematocrit \tag{2.9}$$

$$TBV = Body\,weight * 0.07ml \tag{2.10}$$

TBV—total blood volume.

Erythrocytapheresis is generally safe procedure. However, VA complications can occur; citrate side effects are also possible.

RBC exchange requires additional hydration prior to the procedure. Similarly to erythrocytapheresis, VA and anticoagulant adverse events are possible [74]. Additionally, the patients are exposed to a large HLA antigen pool, increasing the risk for HLA sensitization.

Leukocytapheresis

Leukocytapheresis (LCA) is a procedure, aimed at reducing white blood cell (WBC) count in hyperleukocytosis, a condition characterized by WBC count >100 10^9/L and detected in acute lymphoblastic/myeloid leukemias. Hyperleukocytosis can cause leukostasis, further complicated with hyperviscosity syndrome, vascular occlusions, respiratory failure, and intracranial hemorrhages.

LCA is based on removing WBC by centrifugation, causing WBC depletion. A drop by 10–70% in WBC is aimed in a single procedure.

- Technically, though peripheral VA is preferred, CVC may be needed in many situations, due to patient instability [75]. The procedure should be performed in specialized centers [76]. Citrate is the preferred anticoagulant. Usually, 1.5 up to 2 TBV are processed. The usual WBC volume removed in a single LCA ranges between 200and 1000 ml. Human albumin substitution is warranted if WBC volume removed is more than 20% of TBV.
- Indication: hyperleukocytosis and leukostasis in acute leukemias, currently categorized as ASFA category 3.

- Frequency of LCA: daily, until symptoms of leukostasis disappear.
- Adverse reactions: citrate associated; bleeding, RBC, and PLT loss; VA associated.

Additionally, novel and more specific apheresis methods, processing WBC were developed:

Adsorptive cytapheresis In adsorptive cytapheresis (ACP), a special filter is used to adsorb certain cell populations. Technically, the blood is drawn from the patient; it flows into specialized filter absorbing certain WBC (granulocytes, monocytes, lymphocytes, and platelets). Afterward, the blood is returned to the patient. After removal of inflammatory cells, inflammatory mediators are downregulated; thus, inflammatory process is being suppressed. Three types of filters were developed so far [77]:

1. Cellulose diacetate (AdacolumnTM, JIMRO, Takasaki, Japan): the column is used for adsorbing granulocytes and monocytes.
2. Non-woven polyester fibers (Cellsorba, Asahi Kasei Kuraray Medical, Tokyo, Japan): adsorption of monocytes, granulocytes, lymphocytes, PLT.
3. Polyarylate resin bead (NIKKISO Co., Ltd. Tokyo, Japan): adsorption of monocytes, granulocytes, lymphocytes, PLT.

Generally, the procedure requires peripheral VA. Procedures are performed once or twice weekly, up to 10 ACPs are needed. Biological therapy can be used together with AC.

- Indication: Ulcerative colitis and Crohn disease (especially resistant to biological treatment).
- Adverse events: infection, anticoagulation associated. VA associated; nausea, lymphopenia, concomitant use of ACE inhibitors may cause flushing and hypotension (AdacolumnTM, JIMRO, Takasaki, Japan). ACP demonstrated better safety profile, compared to steroids, immunomodulators, and biological agents [78].

Extracorporeal photopheresis (ECP) Extracorporeal photopheresis is based on centrifugal leukocytapheresis. After centrifugation-based separation of the WBC, they are treated with 8-methoxypsoralen, which is added to the effluent. Separated WBC, treated with 8-methoxypsoralen, are exposed to ultraviolet A (UVA) light and are returned to the patient. The mechanism of action of ECP is not fully determined; however, immunomodulation, induction of apoptosis in certain cell populations, and changes in cytokine synthesis have been suggested [79].

- Technical issues: Peripheral VA is usually needed; CVC is used in more complicated cases. Double needle and single needle methods were used in practice. Both heparin and citrate can be used for anticoagulation. Volume in ECP varies: in adults, processed blood volume ranges from 1.5 to 10 L, depending on the type of ECP (in-line vs. off-line); in children, smaller volumes are used to avoid hypotension [80].
- Two variants exist. In-line ECP performs WBC sequestration, 8-methoxypsoralen treatment, UVA irradiation, and reinfusion in a single device; off-line ECP is performed by two separate devices, the first performs cell separation, whereas the second performs 8-methoxypsoralen treatment and UVA irradiation. The two variants have equal effectiveness.
- Treatment scheme: Usually 2 procedures are performed on 2 consecutive days, which represents 1 cycle. One cycle is performed every 2–4 weeks; however, different protocols were suggested for different diseases.
- Indications: cutaneous T cell lymphoma, graft versus host disease (GVHD), acute rejection in solid organ transplantation (liver, heart, lung).
- Adverse events: anemia, PLT reduction, transient hypotension; ECP does *not* increase the risk for infections.

Thrombocytapheresis

In thrombocytapheresis (TCA), or therapeutic plateletpheresis, PLT are being separated from whole blood by centrifugation.

High PLT counts in essential thrombocytopenia or myeloproliferative neoplasms can cause thrombosis/hemorrhage and ischemia (central nervous system, cardiovascular system). TCA effectively reduces PLT count and ameliorates symptoms [81].

- Technical issues: Usually 1.5–2 TPV are being treated. Peripheral VA is preferred, yet CVC can also be used. Anticoagulation used is citrate or heparin.
- Indication: symptomatic thrombocytosis.
- Treatment schedule: procedures are usually performed daily; PLT count should drop by 30–50% after each TCA. Long-term goal is normalized PLT count. Cytoreductive therapy is needed.
- Adverse events: VA-associated, anticoagulant-associated, hypotension.

Clinical Effectiveness of Therapeutic Apheresis

Clinical effectiveness of different therapeutic apheresis modalities varies across different diseases. In certain cases, PEX was found to have significant impact on disease activity and affects patients survival (acute myasthenia gravis, thrombotic thrombocytopenic purpura, catastrophic antiphospholipid syndrome); in other diseases, PEX had no clear benefit (IgA nephropathy, psoriasis). The American Society for Apheresis (ASFA) has established four distinct categories according to the therapeutic benefit of different apheresis techniques [27]:

- Category I—apheresis is accepted as first-line therapy, either as a primary standalone treatment or in conjunction with other modes of treatment, e.g., PEX for thrombotic thrombocytopenic purpura and lipid apheresis for homozygous familial hypercholesterolemia.
- Category II—apheresis is accepted as second-line therapy, either as a standalone treatment or in conjunction with other modes of treatment, e.g., lipoprotein apheresis in heterozygous

familial hypercholesterolemia, PEX for cryoglobulinemia, and IA for dilated idiopathic cardiomyopathy.
- Category III—Optimum role of apheresis therapy is not established. Decision-making should be individualized, e.g., PEX in IgA nephropathy and PEX for dilated idiopathic cardiomyopathy.
- Category IV—Disorders in which published evidence demonstrates or suggests apheresis to be ineffective or harmful, e.g., PEX for Quinine-induced thrombotic microangiopathy.

In clinical practice, the effect of PEX is evaluated, based on the resolution of clinical symptoms, improvement of laboratory findings, and the effective reduction of target molecule's levels in plasma.

PEX Team Requirements

In order to provide maximum safety and optimize effectiveness, the following recommendations have been published by the German society for transfusion medicine and immunohematology, concerning the practice of the apheresis team [82]:

- Different medical specialties can perform PEX and other apheresis techniques.
- The team (physicians and nurses) should be experienced in extracorporeal techniques.
- The team should be educated in emergency medicine.
- Specific training for each apheresis system is required.
- The team should have at least ten apheresis treatments per system.
- The team should NOT perform more than two apheresis procedures simultaneously.
- The physician should inform the patient about the procedure.
- Written consent is required.
- Personnel's training should be continuously updated.

PEX in Specific Populations

PEX in Children

- Provide space for accompanying person.
- Designated team is required.
- The team is regarded as experienced if at least five apheresis procedures in children have been performed [82].
- Specific training in pediatric emergency medicine/cardiopulmonary resuscitation is required.
- In children with body weight $<$ 20 kg or extracorporeal apheresis system volume exceeds 10% of the total blood volume, priming with cross-matched pre-heated packed red blood cell concentrate/human albumin is recommended.
- Adverse events may present differently, compared to adults.
- Monitor heart rate, oxygen saturation, and blood pressure.
- Peripheral venous lines are preferred, though central lines may be needed. In these cases, the lumen should be tailored to the size of the child (e.g., body weight to 6 kg—dual-lumen 7 French catheter; body weight $>$ 30 kg—dual lumen 10 French catheter) [83].
- Membrane PEX may be preferred due to lower extracorporeal volume (lines and filter, up to 94 ml), compared to cPEX (extracorporeal volume 100–185 ml).
- Plasma volume estimation—different approaches exist; nomograms can be used, but also simplified equation has been suggested [83]:

$$EPV = k^{*} BW^{*} \left(1 - Hct\right) \tag{2.11}$$

EPV—estimated plasma volume, *BW*—body weight, *Hct*—hematocrit, *k*—constant number, measured in ml/kg; k is around 80–90 ml/kg for term infants, 70–75 ml/kg for children, 70 ml/kg for adolescent boys and 65 ml/kg for adolescent girls.

PEX in Pregnancy

- Please note small number of studies, low evidence.
- Generally, PEX is safe in pregnancy; its safety profile is comparable to non-pregnant population.
- Due to removal of clotting factors, provide at least 24 h between last PEX and delivery.
- Blood pressure drop during PEX is more frequently detected in pregnant patients [84].
- Allergic reactions are associated with FFP substitution [84].
- No significant changes in fetal circulation were detected.
- A major obstacle to adequate PEX is calculating the treatment volume in order to achieve 1–1.5 EPV. Due to the increased blood volume in pregnancy, several methods were suggested to correct treatment volume (e.g., increase of EPV by 50% in the last 2 trimesters). However, patient tolerability remains the major determinant in pregnancy.
- Peripheral venous line is preferred; central line may be required in certain cases.

References

1. Cervantes CE, Bloch EM, Sperati CJ. Therapeutic plasma exchange: core curriculum 2023. Am J Kidney Dis. 2023;81(4):475–92. https://doi.org/10.1053/j.ajkd.2022.10.017.
2. Levy JPCD. Plasma exchange. In: Floege J, Johnson R, Feehaly J, editors. Comprehensive clinical nephrology. 4th ed. Philadelphia: Elsevier Saunders; 2010. p. 1108–16.
3. Bambauer R, Latza R, Schiel R. Methods. In: Therapeutic plasma exchange and selective plasma separation methods: fundamental technologies, pathophysiology, and clinical results. 4th ed. Frankfurt\Lengerich: Pabst Science Publisher; 2013. p. 51–191.
4. Deppisch R, Storr M, Buck R, Göhl H. Blood material interactions at the surfaces of membranes in medical applications. Sep Purif Technol. 1998;14(1–3):241–54. https://doi.org/10.1016/S1383-5866(98)00079-3.
5. Ghasemi-Mobarakeh L, Kolahreez D, Ramakrishna S, Williams D. Key terminology in biomaterials and biocompatibility. Curr Opin Biomed Eng. 2019;10:45–50. https://doi.org/10.1016/j.cobme.2019.02.004.

6. BrÜCk SD. Polymeric materials: current status of biocompatibility. Biomater Med Devices Artif Organs. 1973;1(1):79–98. https://doi.org/10.3109/10731197309118864.
7. Canaud B. Recent advances in dialysis membranes. Curr Opin Nephrol Hypertens. 2021;30(6):613–22. https://doi.org/10.1097/MNH.0000000000000744.
8. Weryński A, Malchesky PS, Lewandowski JJ, Waniewski J, Wójcicki J, Piatkiewicz W. Theoretical formulation of sieving coefficient evaluation for membrane plasma separation. Artif Organs. 1985;9(3):250–4. https://doi.org/10.1111/j.1525-1594.1985.tb04387.x.
9. Ahmed S, Kaplan A. Therapeutic plasma exchange using membrane plasma separation. Clin J Am Soc Nephrol. 2020;15(9):1364–70. https://doi.org/10.2215/CJN.12501019.
10. Malchesky PS. Membrane processes for plasma separation and plasma fractionation: guiding principles for clinical use. Ther Apher. 2001;5(4):270–82. https://doi.org/10.1046/j.1526-0968.2001.00337.x.
11. Dehghan R, Barzin J, Carbonell RG, Ghaderi Jafarbeigloo H, Kordkatooli Z. Dextran sulfate bulk and surface-modified microfiltration membrane for simultaneous blood plasma harvesting and low-density lipoprotein removal during plasmapheresis. J Memb Sci. 2024;699:122648. https://doi.org/10.1016/j.memsci.2024.122648.
12. Jaffin MY, Gupta BB, Ding LH, Garreau M. Effect of membrane dimensions and shear rate on plasma filtration for hollow fibres. Trans Am Soc Artif Intern Organs. 1984;30:401–5.
13. Janssens ME, Wakelin S. Centrifugal and membrane therapeutic plasma exchange—a mini-review. Eur Oncol Haematol. 2018;14(2):105–9. https://doi.org/10.17925/EOH.2018.14.2.105.
14. Michel T, Ksouri H, Schneider AG. Continuous renal replacement therapy: understanding circuit hemodynamics to improve therapy adequacy. Curr Opin Crit Care. 2018;24(6):455–62. https://doi.org/10.1097/MCC.0000000000000545.
15. Ejaz AA, Komorski RM, Ellis GH, Munjal S. Extracorporeal circuit pressure profiles during continuous venovenous haemofiltration. Nurs Crit Care. 2007;12(2):81–5. https://doi.org/10.1111/j.1478-5153.2006.00192.x.
16. Elali I, Phachu D, Coombs N, Shah M, Dean J, Haider L, et al. Membrane-based therapeutic plasma exchange: proposed techniques for preventing filter failure. J Clin Apher. 2023;38(5):555–61. https://doi.org/10.1002/jca.22065.
17. Hafer C, Golla P, Gericke M, Eden G, Beutel G, Schmidt JJ, et al. Membrane versus centrifuge-based therapeutic plasma exchange: a randomized prospective crossover study. Int Urol Nephrol. 2016;48(1):133–8. https://doi.org/10.1007/s11255-015-1137-3.
18. Hans R, Tiewsoh K, Lamba DS, Dawman L, Prakash S, Tripathi PP, et al. Centrifugal therapeutic plasma exchange in pediatric patients. Indian J

Pediatr. 2021;88(8):757–63. https://doi.org/10.1007/s12098-020-03657-6.
19. Bustos BR, Hickmann OL, Cruces RP, Díaz F. Therapeutic plasma exchange in critically ill children: experience of the pediatric intensive care unit of two centers in Chile. Transfus Apher Sci. 2021;60(5):103181. https://doi.org/10.1016/j.transci.2021.103181.
20. Webb TN, Bell J, Griffin R, Dill L, Gurosky C, Askenazi D. Retrospective analysis comparing complication rates of centrifuge vs membrane-based therapeutic plasma exchange in the pediatric population. J Clin Apher. 2022;37(3):263–72. https://doi.org/10.1002/jca.21969.
21. Chuang G-T, Huang H-X, Tseng M-H, Tsai I-J, Tsau Y-K. Therapeutic plasma exchange in pediatrics: an overview from the pediatric nephrologists' perspective. Pediatr Neonatol. 2025;66(Suppl 1):S23–7. https://doi.org/10.1016/j.pedneo.2025.01.002.
22. Elhagrasy MAM, El Sayed HM, Emara AA, Abdel-Samea NHA MS. Membrane versus centrifuge based therapeutic plasma exchange. QJM An Int J Med. 2024;117(suppl 2):hcae175.433. https://doi.org/10.1093/qjmed/hcae175.433.
23. Williams ME, Balogun RA. Principles of separation: indications and therapeutic targets for plasma exchange. Clin J Am Soc Nephrol. 2014;9(1):181–90. https://doi.org/10.2215/CJN.04680513.
24. Derksen RHWM, Schuurman HJ, Meyling FHJG, Struyvenberg A, Kater L. The efficacy of plasma exchange in the removal of plasma components. J Lab Clin Med. 1984;104(3):346–54.
25. Winters JL. Plasma exchange: concepts, mechanisms, and an overview of the American Society for Apheresis guidelines. Hematology Am Soc Hematol Educ Program. 2012;1:7–12. https://doi.org/10.1182/asheducation.V2012.1.7.3797920.
26. Kaplan AA. Therapeutic plasma exchange: core curriculum 2008. Am J Kidney Dis. 2008;52(6):1180–96. https://doi.org/10.1053/j.ajkd.2008.02.360.
27. Connelly-Smith L, Alquist CR, Aqui NA, Hofmann JC, Klingel R, Onwuemene OA, et al. Guidelines on the use of therapeutic apheresis in clinical practice—evidence-based approach from the writing Committee of the American Society for apheresis: the ninth special issue. J Clin Apher. 2023;38(2):77–278. https://doi.org/10.1002/jca.22043.
28. Filipov J, Zlatkov B, Emil D, Dimitrov M, Metodieva T, Petrova M, Hristova L, Genov D, Stamenova V. Harakteristika na uslojneniata pri provejdane na plazmafereza v klinika po nefrologia i transplantacia na UMBAL Alexandrovska. Nefrol Dial Transplant. 2015;21:10–5.
29. Goto H, Matsuo H, Nakane S, Izumoto H, Fukudome T, Kambara C, et al. Plasmapheresis affects T helper type-1/T helper type-2 balance of circulating peripheral lymphocytes. Ther Apher. 2001;5(6):494–6. https://doi.org/10.1046/j.1526-0968.2001.00386.x.

30. Hirano R, Namazuda K, Hirata N. Double filtration plasmapheresis: review of current clinical applications. Ther Apher Dial. 2021;25(2):145–51. https://doi.org/10.1111/1744-9987.13548.
31. Ohkubo A, Okado T. Selective plasma exchange. Transfus Apher Sci. 2017;56(5):657–60. https://doi.org/10.1016/j.transci.2017.08.010.
32. Osawa I, Goto T, Kudo D, Hayakawa M, Yamakawa K, Kushimoto S, et al. Targeted therapy using polymyxin B hemadsorption in patients with sepsis: a post-hoc analysis of the JSEPTIC-DIC study and the EUPHRATES trial. Crit Care. 2023;27:245. https://doi.org/10.1186/s13054-023-04533-3.
33. Mitzner S, Kogelmann K, Ince C, Molnár Z, Ferrer R, Nierhaus A. Adjunctive Hemoadsorption therapy with CytoSorb in patients with septic/Vasoplegic shock: a best practice consensus statement. J Clin Med. 2023;12(23):7199. https://doi.org/10.3390/jcm12237199.
34. Schossee N, Veit G, Gittel J, Viebahn J, Niklaus M, Klingler P, et al. Profile of the single-use, multiple-pass protein a adsorber column in immunoadsorption. Vox Sang. 2022;117(3):393–8. https://doi.org/10.1111/vox.13205.
35. Hamilton P, Harris R, Mitra S. Immunoadsorption techniques and its current role in the intensive care unit [Internet]. In: Aspects in continuous renal replacement therapy. IntechOpen; 2019. Available from:. https://doi.org/10.5772/intechopen.84890.
36. Fuchs K, Rummler S, Ries W, Helmschrott M, Selbach J, Ernst F, et al. Performance, clinical effectiveness, and safety of immunoadsorption in a wide range of indications. Ther Apher Dial. 2022;26(1):229–41. https://doi.org/10.1111/1744-9987.13663.
37. Shibuya N, Sato T, Osame M, Takegami T, Doi S, Kawanami S. Immunoadsorption therapy for myasthenia gravis. J Neurol Neurosurg Psychiatry. 1994;57(5):578–81. https://doi.org/10.1136/jnnp.57.5.578.
38. Sugimoto K, Yamaji K, Yang KS, Kanai Y, Tsuda H, Hashimoto H. Immunoadsorption plasmapheresis using a phenylalanine column as an effective treatment for lupus nephritis. Ther Apher Dial. 2006;10(2):187–92. https://doi.org/10.1111/j.1744-9987.2006.00362.x.
39. Suzuki K. The role of immunoadsorption using dextran-sulfate cellulose columns in the treatment of systemic lupus erythematosus. Ther Apher. 2000;4(3):239–43. https://doi.org/10.1046/j.1526-0968.2000.00178.x.
40. Handisurya A, Worel N, Rabitsch W, Bojic M, Pajenda S, Reindl-Schwaighofer R, et al. Antigen-specific Immunoadsorption with the Glycosorb® ABO Immunoadsorption system as a novel treatment modality in pure red cell aplasia following major and bidirectional ABO-incompatible allogeneic hematopoietic stem cell transplantation. Front Med. 2020;7:585628. https://doi.org/10.3389/fmed.2020.585628.
41. Feingold KR. Lipoprotein apheresis. In: Feingold KR, Anawalt B, Blackman MR, et al. editors. Endotext [Internet]. South Dartmouth:

MDText.com, Inc.; 2000–2023. Available from: https://www.ncbi.nlm.nih.gov/books/NBK425700/
42. Miao J, Krisanapan P, Tangpanithandee S, Thongprayoon C, Mao MA, Cheungpasitporn W. Efficacy of extracorporeal plasma therapy for adult native kidney patients with primary FSGS: a systematic review. Ren Fail. 2023;45(1):2176694. https://doi.org/10.1080/0886022X.2023.2176694.
43. Taylan C, Weber LT. An update on lipid apheresis for familial hypercholesterolemia. Pediatr Nephrol. 2023;38(2):371–82. https://doi.org/10.1007/s00467-022-05541-1.
44. Bambauer R, Bambauer C, Lehmann B, Latza R, Schiel R. LDL-apheresis: technical and clinical aspects. Sci World J. 2012;2012:314283. https://doi.org/10.1100/2012/314283.
45. Krieter DH, Jeyaseelan J, Rüth M, Lemke HD, Wanner C, Drechsler C. Clinical hemocompatibility of double-filtration lipoprotein apheresis comparing polyethersulfone and ethylene-vinyl alcohol copolymer membranes. Artif Organs. 2021;45(9):1104–13. https://doi.org/10.1111/aor.13944.
46. Kosmadakis G. Rheopheresis: a narrative review. Int J Artif Organs. 2022;45(5):445–54. https://doi.org/10.1177/03913988221086597.
47. Özdemir ZN, Şahin U, Yıldırım Y, Kaya CT, İlhan O. Lipoprotein apheresis efficacy and challenges: single center experience. Hematol Transfus Cell Ther. 2022;44(1):56–62. https://doi.org/10.1016/j.htct.2021.01.009.
48. Sanchez AP, Ward DM, Cunard R. Therapeutic plasma exchange in the intensive care unit: rationale, special considerations, and techniques for combined circuits. Ther Apher Dial. 2022;26(S1):41–52. https://doi.org/10.1111/1744-9987.13814.
49. Hanaoka A, Naganuma T, Kabata D, Morii D, Takemoto Y, Uchida J, et al. Safety and efficacy of tandem hemodialysis and selective plasma exchange in pretransplant desensitization of ABO-incompatible kidney transplantation. Blood Purif. 2021;50(6):829–36. https://doi.org/10.1159/000512713.
50. Pérez-Sez MJ, Toledo K, Ojeda R, Crespo R, Soriano S, Álvarez De Lara MA, et al. Tandem plasmapheresis and hemodialysis: efficacy and safety. Ren Fail. 2011;33(8):765–9. https://doi.org/10.3109/0886022X.2011.599912.
51. Kumar Mandal A, Garlapati P, Tiongson B, Gayam V. Liver assist devices for liver failure [Internet]. In: Liver pathology. IntechOpen; 2021. https://doi.org/10.5772/intechopen.91287.
52. Rademacher S, Oppert M, Jörres A. Artificial extracorporeal liver support therapy in patients with severe liver failure. Expert Rev Gastroenterol Hepatol. 2011;5(5):591–9. https://doi.org/10.1586/egh.11.59.
53. Barth D, Sanchez A, Thomsen AM, Garcia A, Malachowski R, Weldon R, et al. Peripheral vascular access for therapeutic plasma exchange: a practical approach to increased utilization and selecting the most appropriate

vascular access. J Clin Apher. 2020;35(3):178–87. https://doi.org/10.1002/jca.21778.

54. Mustieles MJ, Lozano M. Vascular access for apheresis: state of the art. Transfus Apher Sci. 2023;62(2):103669. https://doi.org/10.1016/j.transci.2023.103669.
55. Gallieni M, Hollenbeck M, Inston N, Kumwenda M, Powell S, Tordoir J, et al. Clinical practice guideline on peri- and postoperative care of arteriovenous fistulas and grafts for haemodialysis in adults. Nephrol Dial Transplant. 2019;34(Suppl 2):ii1–ii42. https://doi.org/10.1093/ndt/gfz072.
56. Zingg W, Barton A, Bitmead J, Eggimann P, Pujol M, Simon A, et al. Best practice in the use of peripheral venous catheters: a scoping review and expert consensus. Infect Prev Pract. 2023;5(2):100271. https://doi.org/10.1016/j.infpip.2023.100271.
57. Golsorkhi M, Azarfar A, Abdipour A. Vascular access in therapeutic apheresis: one size does not fit all. Ther Apher Dial. 2022;26(4):694–716. https://doi.org/10.1111/1744-9987.13799.
58. Williams LA, Arnesen C, Gunn C, Boshell MN, Pham HP, Guillory B, et al. New subcutaneous PowerFlow port results in cost and time-savings in a busy outpatient apheresis clinic. J Clin Apher. 2019;34:482–6. https://doi.org/10.1002/jca.21678.
59. Doggett BM, Session-Augustine N, Roig J, Strunk M, Valiyaparambil S, Sarode R, et al. Single-needle: an effective alternative to dual-needle peripheral access in therapeutic plasma exchange. J Clin Apher. 2019;34(1):21–5. https://doi.org/10.1002/jca.21665.
60. Shunkwiler SM, Pham HP, Wool G, Ipe TS, Fang DC, Biller E, et al. The management of anticoagulation in patients undergoing therapeutic plasma exchange: a concise review. J Clin Apher. 2018;33(3):371–9. https://doi.org/10.1002/jca.21592.
61. Lee G, Arepally GM. Anticoagulation techniques in apheresis: from heparin to citrate and beyond. J Clin Apher. 2012;27(3):117–25. https://doi.org/10.1002/jca.21222.
62. Kissling S, Legallais C, Pruijm M, Teta D, Vogt B, Burnier M, et al. A new prescription model for regional citrate anticoagulation in therapeutic plasma exchanges. BMC Nephrol. 2017;18(1):81. https://doi.org/10.1186/s12882-017-0494-9.
63. Assefi M, Leurent A, Blanchard F, Quemeneur C, Deransy R, Monsel A, et al. Impact of increasing post-filter ionized calcium target on filter lifespan in renal replacement therapy with regional citrate anticoagulation: a before-and-after study. J Crit Care. 2023;78:154364. https://doi.org/10.1016/j.jcrc.2023.154364.
64. Weinstein R. Prevention of citrate reactions during therapeutic plasma exchange by constant infusion of calcium gluconate with the return fluid. J Clin Apher. 1996;11(4):204–10. https://doi.org/10.1002/(SICI)1098-1101(1996)11:4<204::AID-JCA5>3.0.CO;2-F.

65. Kaplan A, Raut P, Totoe G, Morgan S, Zantek ND. Management of systemic unfractionated heparin anticoagulation during therapeutic plasma exchange. J Clin Apher. 2016;31(6):507–15. https://doi.org/10.1002/jca.21441.
66. Baharoglu MI, Cordonnier C, RAS S, de Gans K, Koopman MM, Brand A, et al. Platelet transfusion versus standard care after acute stroke due to spontaneous cerebral haemorrhage associated with antiplatelet therapy (PATCH): a randomised, open-label, phase 3 trial. Lancet. 2016;387(10038):2605–13. https://doi.org/10.1016/S0140-6736(16)30392-0.
67. Norda R, Stegmayr BG, Berlin G, Kurkus J, Jonsson S, Söderström T, et al. Therapeutic apheresis in Sweden: update of epidemiology and adverse events. Transfus Apher Sci. 2003;29(2):159–66. https://doi.org/10.1016/S1473-0502(03)00121-6.
68. Mafra MP, Roca Mora MM, Godoi A, Valenzuela A. Cryoprecipitate-poor plasma instead of fresh frozen plasma as replacement therapy in thrombotic thrombocytopenic purpura: a systematic review and meta-analysis. Blood. 2023;142(Supplement 1):2629. https://doi.org/10.1182/blood-2023-188500.
69. Kaplan AA. A simple and accurate method for prescribing plasma exchange. ASAIO Trans [Internet]. 1990;36:M597–9. Available from: http://www.ncbi.nlm.nih.gov/entrez/query.fcgi?cmd=Retrieve&db=PubMed&dopt=Citation&list_uids=2252761
70. Floege J, Jayne DRW, Sanders JSF, Tesar V, Rovin BH. KDIGO 2024 clinical practice guideline for the management of Antineutrophil Cytoplasmic Antibody (ANCA)–associated Vasculitis. Kidney Int. 2024;105(3S):S71–S116. https://doi.org/10.1016/j.kint.2023.10.008.
71. Coppo P, Bubenheim M, Azoulay E, Galicier L, Malot S, Bigé N, et al. A regimen with caplacizumab, immunosuppression, and plasma exchange prevents unfavorable outcomes in immune-mediated TTP. Blood. 2021;137(6):733–42. https://doi.org/10.1182/blood.2020008021.
72. Kolonko A, Słabiak-Błaż N, Karkoszka H, Więcek A, Piecha G. The preliminary results of bortezomib used as a primary treatment for an early acute antibody-mediated rejection after kidney transplantation—a single-center case series. J Clin Med. 2020;9(2):529. https://doi.org/10.3390/jcm9020529.
73. Stussi G, Buser A, Holbro A. Red blood cells: exchange, transfuse, or deplete. Transfus. Med. Hemotherapy. 2019;46(6):407–16. https://doi.org/10.1159/000504144.
74. Swerdlow PS. Red cell exchange in sickle cell disease. Hematol Am Soc Hematol Educ Program. 2006:48–53. https://doi.org/10.1182/asheducation-2006.1.48.
75. Aqui N, O'Doherty U. Leukocytapheresis for the treatment of hyperleukocytosis secondary to acute leukemia. Hematol (United States). 2014;2014(1):457–60. https://doi.org/10.1182/asheducation-2014.1.457.

76. Hölig K, Moog R. Leukocyte depletion by therapeutic leukocytapheresis in patients with leukemia. Transfus Med Hemother. 2012;39(4):241–5. https://doi.org/10.1159/000341805.
77. Endo Y, Yonekawa M, Kukita K, Katagiri M, Matsumoto T, Kawasaki K, et al. Novel adsorptive type apheresis device Immunopure for ulcerative colitis from clinical perspectives based on clinical trials: Japan and Europe. Ther Apher Dial. 2021;25(4):432–6. https://doi.org/10.1111/1744-9987.13661.
78. Vernia F, Viscido A, Latella G. Adsorptive cytapheresis in ulcerative colitis: a non-pharmacological therapeutic approach revisited. J Clin Apher. 2023;38(6):746–54. https://doi.org/10.1002/jca.22091.
79. Knobler R, Berlin G, Calzavara-Pinton P, Greinix H, Jaksch P, Laroche L, et al. Guidelines on the use of extracorporeal photopheresis. J Eur Acad Dermatol Venereol. 2014;28(Suppl 1):1–37. https://doi.org/10.1111/jdv.12311.
80. Cid J, Carbassé G, Suárez-Lledó M, Moreno DF, Martínez C, Gutiérrez-García G, et al. Efficacy and safety of one-day offline extracorporeal photopheresis schedule processing one total blood volume for treating patients with graft-versus-host disease. Transfusion. 2019;59(8):2636–42. https://doi.org/10.1111/trf.15384.
81. Zikou X, Vaia D, Vasiliki P, Panagiotis C, Stavros A. Use of therapeutic apheresis methods in ICU. Transfus Apher Sci. 2024;63(1):103853. https://doi.org/10.1016/j.transci.2023.103853.
82. Worel N, Mansouri Taleghani B, Strasser E. Recommendations for therapeutic apheresis by the section "preparative and therapeutic Hemapheresis" of the German society for transfusion medicine and immunohematology. Transfus. Med. Hemotherapy. 2019;46(6):394–406. https://doi.org/10.1159/000503937.
83. Chuang GT, Huang HX, Tseng MH, Tsai IJ, Tsau YK. Therapeutic plasma exchange in pediatrics: an overview from the pediatric nephrologists' perspective. Pediatr Neonatol [Internet]. 2025;66:S23–7. https://doi.org/10.1016/j.pedneo.2025.01.002.
84. Wind M, Gaasbeek AGA, Oosten LEM, Rabelink TJ, van Lith JMM, Sueters M, et al. Therapeutic plasma exchange in pregnancy: a literature review. Eur J Obstet Gynecol Reprod Biol. 2021;260:29–36. https://doi.org/10.1016/j.ejogrb.2021.02.027.

Indications for PEX: Nephrology

3

Abstract

Autoimmune mechanisms are involved in the pathogenesis of broad spectrum of renal diseases. Kidney involvement is due to both primary and secondary glomerular disease in native kidneys. Non-immunological causes can inflict serious damage to the kidneys too (e.g., multiple myeloma). In these cases, the efficacy of PEX and other types of apheresis (e.g., immunoadsorption) have been evaluated, in combination with immunosuppressive therapy. Additionally, PEX has been used in kidney transplantation for the management of antibody-mediated rejection and in desensitization protocols. This chapter will present current body of evidence for the effectiveness of PEX in nephrology.

Keywords

Focal segmental glomerulosclerosis · Anti-glomerular basement membrane disease · Kidney transplantation · Desensitization protocols · Antibody-mediated rejection

J. J. Filipov, *Therapeutic Plasma Exchange*, In Clinical Practice,
https://doi.org/10.1007/978-3-032-17275-4_3

Primary Minimal Change Disease (MCD)

Definition Minimal change disease (MCD) is a condition associated with nephrotic syndrome and normal histological findings (or minimal mesangial proliferation), lacking immunofluorescence staining (or low-intensity C3/IgM deposits) and significant foot-process effacement on electron microscopy. MCD is the most common glomerular disease in children; its prevalence in adults ranges between 10% and 15% [1].

Pathogenesis Several pathogenic mechanisms for MCD have been suggested: genetic (mutations of slit-diaphragm proteins), humoral (unidentified so far circulating factor), T cell abnormalities, and loss of negative charge of glomerular basement membrane (GBM). Secondary forms, associated with drugs, allergies and neoplasia (especially Hodgkin lymphoma), are also present.

Clinical presentation MCD presents with nephrotic syndrome. The disease is usually steroid-responsive, and generally has good prognosis.

Treatment In most of the cases, steroids effectively achieve remission both in children and in adults. In steroid-resistant cases, additional agents are used [Cyclophosphamide, calcineurin inhibitors (CNI), mycophenolic acid derivatives, Rituximab]. Secondary forms should be ruled out.

PEX in MCD Current guidelines do not suggest the use of PEX in the treatment of MCD [2, 3].

However, a recent study demonstrated the effectiveness of apheresis methods (PEX, LA, IA, DFPP) in refractory idiopatic nephrotic syndrome in native kidneys. The retrospective study included nine patients with MCD. Though the study included heterogeneous group of patients [MCD and focal segmental glomerulosclerosis (FSGS)] and various methods were used, it demonstrated possible benefit from therapeutic plasmapheresis in resistant cases [4].

Additionally, a small study demonstrated benefit from LA in two cases with MCD, presenting with acute kidney injury [5]. Thus, in resistant MCD subjects different therapeutic plasmapheresis techniques can be tried as salvage therapy, applying the therapeutic approach for FSGS (see next section).

Primary Focal Segmental Glomerulosclerosis (FSGS)

Definition Primary FSGS is a syndrome consisting of focal (affecting less than 50% of the glomeruli) segmental (affecting part of glomerular tuft) glomerulosclerosis on light microscopy, diffuse foot-process effacement on electron microscopy, and clinical and laboratory data for nephrotic syndrome (proteinuria >3.5 g/24 h, hypoproteinemia, often presenting with edema, dyslipidemia). Secondary FSGS should be ruled out when the diagnosis is detected on biopsy (viral etiology, drugs, maladaptive changes due to reduced nephron mass or sclerotic changes due to hyperfiltration, without nephron loss), as well as genetic forms (due to mutations of podocyte or glomerular basement membrane proteins). A fourth group of FSGS patients is classified, FSGS of undetermined cause, encompassing most probably undiagnosed genetic or secondary forms [2].

Pathogenesis The etiology of primary FSGS is unclear. Similar pathogenic factors for MCD were suggested for primary FSGS. In FSGS, the role of undetected so far circulating factor has been discussed too, especially in the light of FSGS recurrence after kidney transplantation, where PEX was found to be effective. The relationship between primary MCD and primary FSGS has been discussed over the years, as many researchers regard these two conditions as two forms of a single disease, in which podocyte injury plays a pivotal role.

Clinical presentation Generally, primary FSGS presents with acute onset of nephrotic syndrome with edema. A more insidious course, the presence of nephrotic range proteinuria without nephrotic syndrome or non-nephrotic proteinuria may indicate secondary forms and etiology should be clarified. Genetic testing may be performed too, especially in young adults and children with family history of kidney disease, resistant to treatment [6].

Treatment Initially, secondary FSGS should be excluded. Immunosuppressive treatment is recommended for primary FSGS. Steroids, CNIs were suggested; in frequent relapses,rituximab, cyclophosphamide, mycophenolic acid derivatives can be used [2].

PEX in primary FSGS Plasma exchange, as well as other apheresis modalities—IA and lipoprotein apheresis (LA)—can be used in refractory primary FSGS and in recurrent FSGS after kidney transplantation. PEX/IA/LA can be performed in adults and children [7].

- Drug-resistant FSGS in native kidneys—PEX effectiveness is uncertain; LA can be used as second-line treatment.
- Recurrent FSGS after kidney transplantation—PEX and IA should be used as first-line treatment (ASFA category 1);

except for PEX/IA, additional immunosuppressive agents are used, including novel medications, e.g., ofatumumab and abatacept [8]. PEX/IA should be started as soon as recurrence is confirmed. Both PEX and IA have been used for the prevention of FSGS recurrence after kidney transplantation; however, the effectiveness of this approach requires further evaluation and is not supported by current guidelines [9, 10].

PEX/IA/LA schedule:

- Treatment volume per TA: 1.0–1.5 EPV; regenerative IA: 2.5PV; LA—treatment volume may vary in different types of lipoprotein apheresis.
- Substitution: albumin or FFP (PEX), none in IA and LA.
- Interval between sessions: 24–48 h (PEX), LA—twice weekly for 3 weeks.
- End of treatment: clinical and laboratory improvement; maintenance treatment is also possible, highly individualized.

PEX and other techniques for plasmapheresis are demonstrated in Table 3.1.

Table 3.1 PEX and other plasmapheresis methods in the treatment of FSGS [3, 7, 9]

Condition	Treatment modality	Treatment volume	Substitution fluid	Frequency	Maintenance treatment
Drug-resistant FSGS—native kidney	PEX	1–1.5 EPV	Albumin/FFP	Daily procedure for 3 days	3 procedures for 2–3 weeks[a]
Drug-resistant FSGS—native kidney	LA	1–1.5 EPV	None	2 LA weekly–3 weeks	1 LA weekly–6 weeks
Post-transplant recurrence	PEX	1–1.5 EPV	Albumin/FFP	Daily procedure for 3 days	3 procedures for 2–3 weeks[a]
Post-transplant recurrent FSGS	IA—single use column	1–1.5 EPV	None	Similar to PEX	Similar to PEX
Post-transplant recurrent FSGS	IA—regenerative adsorbers	2–3 EPV	None	Similar to PEX	Similar to PEX
Post-transplant recurrent FSGS	LA	1–1.5 EPV	None	2 LA weekly–3 weeks	1 LA weekly–6 weeks
Prevention of FSGS recurrence (living donor)	PEX	1.5 EPV	Albumin	3 procedures prior to KT 3 procedures every other day post-operatively	
Prevention of FSGS recurrence (deceased donor)	PEX	1.5 EPV	Albumin	3 procedures post-operatively, every other day	

FSGS focal segmental glomerulosclerosis, *PEX* therapeutic plasma exchange, *LA* lipoprotein apheresis, *IA* immunoadsorption, *EPV* estimated plasma volume, *FFP* fresh frozen plasma, [a]maintenance treatment depends on clinical response

Primary Membranous Nephropathy

Definition Membranous nephropathy (MN) is an autoimmune disease, characterized with diffuse or granular immune deposits, consisting of IgG and complement factors, localized beneath the podocytes, on the subepithelial side of the GBM. MN is the most common glomerular disease in adults above 60 years of age; up to 30% of all cases have defined etiology [viral disease (hepatitis B, hepatitis C, HIV), autoimmune disease (SLE), cancers (breast, colon, prostate, bronchi), drugs (nonsteroidal anti-inflammatory drugs, NSAIDs; penicillamine, gold)].

Pathogenesis Primary MN is an autoimmune disease. Several autoantibodies have been identified with MN: anti-phospholipase A2 receptor antibodies (anti-PLA2R-Ab), which is detected in 80% of the cases with primary MN, anti-neutral endopeptidase antibodies (anti-NEP-Ab), and anti-THSD7A antibodies. Other autoantibodies have also been linked to primary MN (e.g., anti-protocadherin 7-Ab, anti-exostosin 1/2-Ab) [11]. Additional factors such as genetic variations and environmental factors can contribute to the development of primary MN.

Clinical presentation MN presents with nephrotic syndrome. However, additional findings may be present—microscopic hematuria, reduced glomerular filtration rate (GFR), and hypertension. Symptoms of systemic disease (SLE, neoplasia) can be observed.

Treatment Prior to initiating treatment, secondary MN should be excluded. The current treatment strategies for MN treatment include supportive care and immunosuppressive therapy (steroids + cyclophosphamide, CNIs, Rituximab, or combination of these medications) [2].

PEX in the treatment of MN Current guidelines do not discuss the use of PEX or other alternative modalities in the treatment of primary MN. Small studies evaluated the effectiveness of PEX/IA for MN.

A study using PEX and RTX or IVIG for rescue treatment in resistant MN achieved partial remission in 10 patients, compared to conservative treatment [12].

Additionally, five daily sessions of peptide GAM-IA demonstrated reduction in anti-PLA2R-Ab in patients with MN. The treatment was well tolerated, but did not achieve reduction in proteinuria [13].

Further evaluation of effectiveness of PEX/IA in primary MN is needed.

Anti-glomerular Basement Membrane (Anti-GBM) Disease

Definition Anti-GBM disease is a rare condition, in which autoantibodies against the glomerular basement membrane (GBM) are formed. A more narrow term Goodpasture's disease defines the presence of antibodies specifically against the non-collagenous domain of α3 chain of collagen type IV. Both conditions present with rapidly progressive glomerulonephritis (RPGN) ± lung hemorrhage. Lung involvement is associated with high mortality. Immunological renal and lung involvement is referred as Goodpasture's syndrome; other etiologies for Goodpasture's syndrome are ANCA vasculitis, SLE—these conditions will be discussed in other sections of this book.

Pathogenesis The mechanism for renal and lung injury are the presence of autoantibodies, aiming different components of the GBM and alveolar basement membrane, most often the α3 chain of collagen type IV. Certain genetic factors and environmental factor may play a role in the pathogenesis. Alveolar hemorrhage is associated with smoking, fluid overload, and pulmonary infection.

Clinical presentation Anti-GBM disease presents with rapidly deteriorating kidney function, hematuria, and oliguria. Symptoms of alveolar hemorrhage include hemoptysis, respiratory failure, and are present in 40–60% of the patients [14]. Lung involvement is diagnosed via CT scan of the lungs; increased uptake of inhaled carbon monoxide is the most sensitive test for alveolar hemorrhage. Kidney biopsy usually reveals crescents, as well as linear IgG deposition on immunofluorescence. Elevated titers of anti-GBM antibodies are present. ANCA antibodies can also be present, which is regarded as a form of anti-GBM disease, linked to faster progression of the disease, with more frequent relapses.

Treatment Immunosuppression should be started as early as possible. Pulse steroids and Cyclophosphamide are the first-line choice; alternatively, in refractory cases, Rituximab and mycophenolate can be used as substitute to Cyclophosphamide.

PEX in the treatment of anti-GBM disease PEX plays a pivotal role in the treatment of the disease. Its role is particularly important in cases with diffuse alveolar hemorrhage (DAH) and those patients, who are not dialysis dependent. However, dialysis-dependent cases at presentation or those with 100% crescents/more than 50% glomerulosclerosis on biopsy may not benefit from PEX and the decision for PEX should take possible side effects into consideration [2].

- DAH (dialysis independent/dependent)—PEX is part of the first-line treatment. ASFA category 1.
- Dialysis independent anti-GBM disease, serum creatinine <5.7 mg/L(503 µmol/L) (no lung involvement)—PEX is first-line treatment, ASFA category 1.
- Dialysis dependent, serum creatinine >5.7 mg/L (503 µmol/L)— consider benefit/harm; ASFA category 3 [3].
- PEX should be performed daily in DAH and every other day in renal anti-GBM disease without lung hemorrhage. Usually 7 to 10 procedures are required.
- Treatment PEX volume is 1.0–1.5 EPV.
- FFP is the substitution fluid in DAH; otherwise, human albumin is used. Treatment is coupled with immunosuppression, aiming at negative ant-GBM serology.
- IA and DFPP also demonstrated effective removal of anti-GBM-Ab.
- End of treatment: clinical and laboratory improvement.

Infection-Associated Glomerular Disease

Definition Infection-associated glomerular disease (IAGD) is linked to different infectious agents:

- Bacterial: *Streptococcus*, *Staphylococcus epidermidis*, Gram /–/ negative bacteria [post-infectious glomerulonephritis (GN), shunt nephritis, endocarditis-related GN, IgA-dominant infection-related GN]
- Viral: hepatitis C (HCV), hepatitis B (HBV), human immunodeficiency virus–related glomerular diseases
- Parasitic: malaria, schistosomiasis, filariasis–associated glomerular diseases

A wide range of histological changes can be observed—endocapillary hypercelularity, membranoproliferative GN, secondary FSGS, secondary membranous nephropathy, and cryoglobulinemic vasculitis [15, 16].

Pathogenesis Different mechanisms for glomerular injury in infection-related glomerulopathies were described—deposition of immune complexes, antigen mimicry, infectious antigen deposition in glomerular structures, and formation of autoantibodies.

Clinical presentation IAGD may present with hematuria, proteinuria, and deterioration of kidney function. The symptoms have different presentation in the different types of IAGD. Active symptoms of the initial infection or history for infection may be present. Systemic involvement may be detected in cryoglobulinemic vasculitis (skin purpura, ulceration of extremities, arthralgia, liver and glomerular involvement, neuropathy, abdominal pain).

Treatment Generally, infection-associated GN requires supportive treatment and etiological treatment. Immunosuppression is not required, it has uncertain impact on disease prognosis and is applied in specific situations. Immunosuppression is required in certain cases of HCV-associated GN (nephrotic range proteinuria, rapidly deteriorating kidney function, cryoglobulinemic flare); in HBV-associated GN, immunosuppression is generally avoided; PEX can be considered in HBV and cryoglobulinemic vasculitis [2, 17].

PEX in the treatment of IAGD PEX use is limited to the cases of HCV and HBV-associated GN, complicated with cryoglobulinemic vasculitis, with/ or without immunosuppression (ASFA category 2). Other apheresis methods can be used too: DFPP, IA; cryofyltration can be applied, but removal of cryoglobulins is poorer, compared to DFPP [3].

- Treatment volume: 1–1.5 EPV.
- Replacement fluid: human albumin.
- Interval between PEX: 24–72 h. 3–8 procedures are suggested and re-evaluation of the patients should be performed. Maintenance PEX/DFPP/IA may be required.
- End of treatment: with resolution of symptoms. Cryocrit is not recommended as marker for initiation or discontinuation of treatment [3].

Membranoproliferative Glomerular Disease (MPGN)

Definition Membranoproliferative glomerulonephritis (MPGN) refers to a specific kidney injury, characterized on light microscopy by increased intraglomerular cells and diffuse thickening of glomerular capillary wall. Immunofluorescence findings are the cornerstone of current classification of MPGN. Basically, three subtypes are present, reflecting different pathogenic mechanisms [2]:

- Immunoglobulin deposition ± complement—kidney injury is mediated by immunoglobulins or immune complexes; major etiology are infections (HCV, HBV, bacterial, protozoa), autoimmune diseases (SLE, mixed connective tissue disease, Sjögren syndrome, Rheumatoid arthritis), monoclonal gammopathies, idiopathic MPGN, and fibrillary glomerulonephritis.

- Complement dominant subgroup—divided further to C3/C4 deposit subtypes—kidney injury is linked to alternative pathway complement activation, due to mutations or antibodies to complement factors or complement regulatory proteins: C3/C4 GN, C3/C4—dense deposit disease.
- Immunofluorescence negative subgroup—associated with thrombotic microangiopathy (TMA), antiphospholipid syndrome, sickle cell anemia, polycytemia vera; polyneuropathy, organomegaly, endocrinopathy, monoclonal protein, and skin changes (POEMS) syndrome.

Clinical presentation MPGN may present with proteinuria, nephrotic syndrome, and hematuria; GFR can be reduced. In more severe cases, the disease may present with rapidly progressive glomerulonephritis, systemic symptoms may be detected secondary MPGN due to autoimmune disease malignancy and infection (HCV, cryoglobulinemia).

Treatment Therapy is focused on underlying condition (infection, neoplasia, autoimmune disease complement dysregulation). Idiopathic MPGN, presenting with nephrotic range proteinuria, active urine sediment, abnormal GFR steroids, and immunosuppressive agents can be considered (mycophenolate, cyclophosphamide, Rituximab). In C3 GN, steroids, mycophenolate, Eculisumab can be used. In cases of rapidly progressive crescentic idiopathic MPGN, immunosuppressive protocol for ANCA-associated vasculitis can be applied [2].

PEX in the treatment of MPGN PEX may be used in certain situations: presence of cryoglobulinemic vasculitis, especially in HCV patients, presence of catastrophic antiphospholipid syndrome (CAPS), and SLE. The apheresis methods will be discussed in the sections for cryoglobulinemia, SLE, and CAPS, respectively.

IgA Nephropathy (IgAN) and IgA Vasculitis (IgAV)

Definition IgAN is the most common form of primary glomerulonephritis and an important cause for CKD worldwide. IgA may present with wide range of histological findings on light microscopy (mesangial proliferation, crescent formation, glomerular sclerosis and interstitial fibrosis/tubular atrophy). Diffuse IgA mesangial deposits are typical for the disease, accompanied by IgG and C3 deposits.

IgAV (previously Henoch-Schönlein Purpura) is a small vessel vasculitis, affecting joints, skin, bowels, kidneys, rarely involving the central nervous system (CNS). IgA deposition in the vessel wall triggers inflammation and organ dysfunction.

Pathogenesis For IgAN, defective glycosylation of IgA1 antibodies, leading to the production of galactose-deficient IgA1 is the initial step. The process has mucosal origin and is influenced by genetic and environmental factors. Antibodies against galactose-deficient IgA1 are formed (IgG, IgA) and immune complexes are formed, which are deposited in the mesangium, starting inflammation. Similar pathogenesis is present in IgAV; immune complexes are deposited in the endothelial cells [18, 19].

Clinical presentation IgAN can present with a wide range of symptoms and laboratory findings: macroscopic hematuria, microscopic hematuria with proteinuria, chronic kidney disease, and rarely acute kidney injury. In IgAV, palpable purpura is characteristic, as well as arthralgia, kidney involvement, abdominal pain ± bloody diarrhea. Rarely CNS involvement may be present [3].

Treatment Supportive care is the first step in IgAN treatment. Steroids can be considered in patients with risk for CKD progression. High-dose steroids and immunosuppressive agents are suggested in rapidly progressive crescentic IgAN. Novel agents, reflecting the improved knowledge of IgAN pathogenesis, are also being implemented in clinical practice. Supportive care is suggested in IgAV; in severe cases, steroids and immunosuppressive therapy can be used [2].

PEX in the treatment of IgAN/IgAV The role of PEX in the treatment of IgAN/IgAV is not fully elucidated. Its use is suggested in crescentic or rapidly progressive IgAN, as well as in severe IgAV, but its effectiveness is uncertain (ASFA category 3). A potential role of PEX is considered if added to steroid treatment in IgA vasculitis with extrarenal manifestations in uncontrolled studies. A potential role of PEX is considered if added to steroid treatment in IgA vasculitis with extrarenal manifestations in uncontrolled studies [20].

- Treatment volume per PEX: 1–1.5 EPV.
- Interval between PEX sessions: 48–72 h.
- Substitution fluid: human albumin/FFP; FFP should be considered in bleeding.
- End of treatment: resolution of symptoms/improvement in kidney function; different maintenance protocols (e.g., 4–11 PEX sessions over 21 days in IgAV) exist [3].

Myeloma Cast Nephropathy

Definition Multiple myeloma (MM) affects the kidney in different mechanisms, leading to a wide spectrum of MM-associated renal injury: MPGN, amyloidosis, Fanconi syndrome, immunotactoid glomerulonephritis, pre-renal acute kidney injury (AKI) due to dehydration, hypercalcemia; myeloma cast nephropathy [21]. The latter is the most common finding and is associated with filtering free light chains (FLC) into the tubules, which react with uromodulin, form protein casts within the distal tubules.

Pathogenesis FLC form aggregates with uromodulin, which cause obstruction of distal tubules and direct proximal tubule nephrotoxicity. Renal damage is further aggravated by loop diuretics, hypercalcemia, dehydration, and infection.

Clinical presentation Myeloma cast nephropathy presents with different stages of AKI; some of the patients may be dialysis dependent. The disease may progress to chronic kidney disease (CKD) too.

Treatment The treatment of myeloma cast nephropathy has two major goals—applying adequate chemotherapy (in order to control MM and reduce FLC) and supportive measures—adequate hydration, avoidance of nephrotoxic agents, correction of hypercalcemia, treatment of urinary tract infections, and renal replacement therapy if needed. Extracorporeal removal of FLC with PEX/hemodialysis (high-cut off) can also be considered.

PEX in the treatment of myeloma cast nephropathy Early reduction in FLC was associated with better survival; however, PEX is a second-line therapy in myeloma cast nephropathy (ASFA category 2). It can be added to chemotherapy (first-line treatment) [3]. High-cut off hemodialysis removes effectively FLC, but has no impact on all-cause mortality and renal outcomes [22].

- Treatment volume per PEX: 1–1.5 EPV
- Substitution fluid: human albumin
- Interval between PEX sessions: 24–48 h; duration 14–28 days
- End of treatment: improvement in kidney function, reduction in FLC ≥50%

Lupus Nephritis

Definition SLE is autoimmune disease, affecting various organs, including the kidneys. Lupus nephritis (LN) affects up to 60% of the patients with SLE and is regarded as life-threatening organ damage. LN has several histological forms.

Pathogenesis Various factors (environmental, humoral, and genetic) can cause production of autoantibodies. They have either direct effect on different organs or cause injury by forming immune complexes in situ or deposited in the renal tissue.

Clinical presentation LN may present with nephrotic syndrome, as well as hematuria (microscopic/macroscopic) and impaired kidney function (AKI/CKD). Systemic findings may also be present (e.g., skin, joints, cardiovascular system). SLE may be complicated with TMA (complement-mediated TMA/thrombotic thrombocytopenic purpura) and catastrophic anti-phospholipid syndrome (cAPS).

Treatment Immunosuppressive protocols, based on steroids, cyclophosphamide, RTX, Belimumab, and mycophenolates have been developed. Eculizumab can be used in LN with complement-mediated TMA [23]. In addition, supportive treatment is used (renal protection, anticoagulants, hypertensive treatment).

PEX in the treatment of LN PEX is currently added to treatment in severe or refractory to treatment SLE, especially complicated with TMA, cAPS, DAH, and progressive LN (ASFA category 2) [2, 23]. More intensive PEX regimen is used for LN and DAH.

- Treatment volume per PEX procedure: 1–1.5 EPV.
- Substitution fluid: human albumin/FFP.
- Interval between PEX sessions: 24–48 h (LN, DAH); 48 h for other complications [3]; 24 h interval for TMA/cAPS with FFP substitution is required.
- End of treatment: clinical improvement.

Kidney Transplantation (KT)

Therapeutic apheresis is used in kidney transplantation in two major aspects: desensitization protocols in AB0 incompatible KT or HLA-sensitized candidates for KT; treatment of antibody-mediated rejection (AbMR) or recurrent glomerular disease after KT.

AB0-Incompatible KT, Living Donor

Definition A- and B antigens are glycoproteins, expressed not only on the surface of RBC, but also on epithelial cells, vascular endothelial cells, and collecting and distal renal tubules. Naturally existing antibodies bind to A/B antigens, triggering complement activation, neutrophil and monocyte infiltration, and damage to target cells (RBC, endothelium, tubular cells) [24].

Pathogenesis Kidney transplant recipient (KTR) antibodies bind to A/B donor antigens, activating the complement, causing severe and rapid damage to vascular endothelium, renal tubules. Hyperacute rejection develops, leading to formation of thrombi of small vessels, endothelial damage, and rapid transplant loss. Therefore, AB0 incompatibility is a serious obstacle to successful KT. Current strategies for desensitization effectively enlarge the donor pool.

Clinical presentation AB0-incompatible (AB0i) KT presents with immediate graft loss after connecting the donor kidney to recipient circulation. These cases are rarely seen due to adequate immunological tests prior to KT. Two major strategies for avoiding hyperacute rejection in AB0-incompatible KT exist: removal of circulating antibodies and immunomodulation; donor exchange [24].

Treatment Antibody removal (therapeutic apheresis), combined with immunomodulation, is the cornerstone of desensitization strategy in AB0-incompatible KT, aiming most commonly at isoagglutinin titers of 1:8. Current desensitization protocols achieve significant improvement in AB0i graft survival. The current immunomodulation is based on Rituximab (RTX), anti-thymocyte globulin (ATG), intravenous immunoglobulins (IVIG); splenectomy is generally not performed. PEX, DFFP, and IA are the options for antibody removal and are first-line option for AB0i candidates (ASFA category 1). CNI and mycophenolates can be started prior to

KT; post-transplant triple immunosuppressive regimen is used. Basiliximab or ATG can be used as induction therapy.

- Treatment volume per TA procedure: 1–1.5 EPV for PEX, DFFP; 2–2.5 EPV for IA
- Substitution: human albumin/FFP (AB0 compatible)
- Interval between PEX sessions: 24–48 h
- End of PEX/IA: after achieving target isoagglutinin titer, depends on transplant center

Several protocols for ABOi KT desensitization are demonstrated in Table 3.2

Table 3.2 Desensitization protocols in AB0i KT [25–27]

Target isoagglutinin titer at day of KT	Apheresis protocol	Immunomodulation	Results
≤1:8/≤1:32	PEX, every other day, Start 7 days prior to KT	RTX 200 mg [day (−15)]; IVIG 5 g after each PEX (total 10–25 g), Thymoglobulin—two doses, day 0 and 1 post KT, total 3 mg/kg	1-year graft and patient survival 97.8%
≤1:8	DFPP: 7 days prior to KT, every other day, performed post KT	RTX [day (−14)] Tacrolimus and mycophenolate initiated at day (−7)	Graft survival 87%, patient survival 93%, Desensitization rate 100%
≤1:8	Antigen-specific IA Start:6 days prior to KT; four sessions, Post-KT: 3 IA over 9 days	RTX 375 mg/m^2 [day (−14)] Immunosuppression (Tac, MMF, CS) started at day (−7) IVIG 0.5 g/kg after final IA	All patients had good graft function during the follow-up

KT kidney transplantation, *PEX* therapeutic plasma exchange, *RTX* rituximab, *DFPP* double filtration plasmapheresis, *IA* immunoadsorption, *Tac* tacrolimus, *MMF* mycophenolate mofetil, *CS* corticosteroids, *IVIG* intravenous immunoglobulin

HLA-Sensitized KT Candidates in AB0-Compatible KT

Definition The presence of donor-specific anti-HLA antibodies is a serious obstacle to KT and graft survival. The major events associated with HLA sensitization are blood products transfusion, pregnancy, previous KT, and graft nephrectomy.

Pathogenesis Anti-HLA donor-specific alloantibodies (DSA) in pre-sensitized recipients bind to donor HLA antigens, causing activation of complement and damage to donor organ.

Clinical presentation Clinically, HLA sensitization presents with acute/hyperacute rejection. Currently, with the regular performance of crossmatch testing prior to KT these cases are extremely rare.

Treatment Desensitization protocols were developed based on antibody removal and immunomodulation. However, current guidelines recommend antibody avoidance (e.g., donor exchange programs) to desensitization [10].

Due to its unclear benefit, desensitization is not recommended candidates for deceased donor KT [3].

In living donation, TPE/IA are coupled with immunomodulation (most commonly Rituximab, IVIG) and immunosuppressive agents (Tacrolimus, mycophenolates), as well as induction with Thymoglobulin. Usually five procedures TPE/IA prior to KT are performed, daily/every other day. Mean fluorescence intensity (MFI) of DSA can be used to choose the type of therapeutic apheresis—PEX in MFI ≤9000, DFFP in MFI ranging between 9000 and 12,000, IA in MFI >12,000 [28]. TPE/IA is first-line treatment in HLA desensitization (ASFA category 1).

- Treatment volume per TA: 1–1.5 EPV (PEX), 2–2.5 EPV (IA).
- Substitution fluid: human albumin. Consider FFP preoperatively.

- Interval between sessions: 24–48 h. Five procedures prior to KT, at least 3 post-transplant.
- End of PEX/IA: achieved negative crossmatch and reduction of MFI to pre-designed levels, specific for each transplant center.

HLA-Sensitized Candidates in AB0-Incompatible KT

Generally, KT in HLA-sensitized, AB0-incompatible candidates is regarded riskier, compared to AB0 incompatibility or HLA sensitization alone [29]. However, in this rare recipient-donor immunological setting, desensitization protocols were developed too. A small study using PEX or specific/nonspecific IA, combined with IVIG, two doses of RTX (375 mg/m^2) and Tacrolimus (0.2 mg/kg started 10 days prior to KT) demonstrated excellent graft and patient survival [30].

Technically, PEX/IA is performed similarly to AB0 incompatible KT and HLA-sensitized recipients—see previous sections of this Chapter.

Treatment of Antibody-Mediated Rejection (AbMR)

Definition Acute/active AbMR is defined by the presence of all three findings [31]:

(a) Histological evidence of tissue injury (at least one of the following: microvascular inflammation, transmural/intimal arteritis, acute thrombotic microangiopathy, acute tubular injury)
(b) Evidence of antibody interaction with vascular endothelium (e.g., C4d linear staining, microvascular inflammation, increased expression of tissue genes for endothelial injury)
(c) Serologic presence of DSA (to HLA/non-HLA antigens)

Chronic active AbMR is defined by the presence of:

(a) Morphologic evidence of chronic tissue injury (transplant, severe peritubular capillary basement membrane multilayering, arterial intimal fibrosis of new onset)
(b) Evidence of current/recent antibody interaction with vascular endothelium
(c) Serologic evidence of DSA (to HLA /non-HLA antigens)

The spectrum of AbMR further encompasses C4d negative AbMR and Ab-mediated vascular rejection (presence of intimal arteritis).

Pathogenesis AbMR is triggered by the presence of DSAs, most commonly targeting HLA antigens. De novo DSAs appear after successful KT. Pre-existing anti-HLA DSAs can also cause AbMR; although successful desensitization protocols are applied (see Sects. 3.9.1 and 3.9.2), donor-specific HLA antigen avoidance is preferred [10]. Antibodies against non-HLA antigens can also trigger AbMR (e.g., MICA, AT1R antigens).

Clinical presentation AbMR usually presents with rapid deterioration of graft function. In the rare cases of hyperacute AbMR, rapid ischemia after connecting the donor nor kidney to the recipient's circulation occurs, resulting in practically instantaneous graft loss. Chronic AbMR has insidious course, presenting with proteinuria and GFR reduction over years post-transplant.

Treatment of AbMR Therapeutic apheresis (PEX/IA) and immunomodulation are the key components of acute AMR. Usually 5 PEX/IA procedures (4–7) are performed; high-dose steroids and IVIG (100–400 mg/kg after each PEX/IA or 2 gr/kg 0 1–4 doses) are the most commonly used immune modulators. Additionally, Rituximab (375 mg/m^2 weekly, 2–4 doses) and bortezomib (1.3–1.5 mg/m^2 × 4 doses) were used, though their effectiveness is inconclusive [32]. The ASFA guidelines place PEX/IA as first-line treatment (ASFA category 1) in acute AbMR in AB0-compatible KT; in AB0i KT PEX/IA are second-line treatment [3]

- Treatment volume per TA procedure: 1–1.5 EPV (PEX), 2–2.5 EPV (IA).
- Substitution fluid: human albumin/FFP.
- Interval between TA procedures: 24–48 h; 4–7 procedures may be required.
- End of PEX/IA: reversal of laboratory and histological findings.

Nephrectomy is the only treatment option in hyperacute AbMR. In chronic active AbMR, PEX/IA has limited benefit due to the chronic histological changes in the graft [33].

Recurrent Glomerular Disease

Recurrent glomerular disease is significant contributor to graft loss. Theoretically, all types of glomerular diseases can recur post-transplant [2].

Recurrent FSGS FSGS recurs in the early post-transplant period. Previous graft loss due to recurrence is regarded as a risk factor for a new episode in the second graft. Treatment protocol, including therapeutic apheresis in recurrent FSGS, has been discussed in section "Primary Focal Segmental Glomerulosclerosis (FSGS)".

Recurrent anti-GBM disease Anti-GBM disease after successful KT is a rare finding and some reports consider immunosuppression withdrawal as possible risk factor for recurrence [34]. A major contributor to low recurrence after KT is the requirement for negative anti-GBM serology for 9–12 months prior to KT

[10]. Treatment of anti-GBM recurrence follows the steps outlined in section "Anti-glomerular Basement Membrane (Anti-GBM) Disease".

Recurrent IgAN/IgAV IgAN/IgAV has relatively high recurrence rates, estimated up to 53%; graft loss was estimated to be 9.7%. Currently, the immunosuppressive strategies had no significant impact on graft survival. The benefit from PEX/IA in recurrent IgAN/IgAV is unclear; the regimen, given in section "IgA Nephropathy (IgAN) and IgA Vasculitis (IgAV)" can be considered with caution.

Recurrent MN Post-transplant MN recurrence peaks up to 55%, with recurrence risk associated with higher titers of anti-PLA2R–Ab [35]. Recurrence incidence increases in the long run. Current treatment suggests the use of RTX in these cases. There is insufficient data to suggest the use of therapeutic apheresis in recurrent MN.

Recurrent MPGN MPGN demonstrated high recurrence rate and high prevalence of graft loss after recurrence. Several risk factors were established in living related donation, low C3/C4 levels, preemptive KT [36]. Earlier reports demonstrated benefit from the use of PEX in recurrent MPGN [37]; however, the findings from more recent papers using PEX ± RTX are controversial, achieving reversal of MPGN in no more than 50% of the cases [36].

Recurrent ANCA-associated vasculitis (AAV) As ANCA-associated vasculitis can relapse after KT, complete clinical remission is required prior to transplantation. Primary AAV is treated with steroids, cyclophosphamide, RTX; though the data for clinical benefit from therapeutic apheresis are inconsistent, it is recommended in cases with poorer kidney function, progressive kidney disease, diffuse alveolar hemorrhage (DAH), as well as refractory cases [38]. Generally, post-transplant AAV relapse is effectively controlled with current immunosuppression [39]. PEX can be used in complicated cases as mentioned in primary AAV. For more details, please refer to section "ANCA-Associated Vasculitis", Chap. 5 of this book.

Recurrent LN Post-transplant LN relapse rate varies and may reach up to 54% [40]. Various risk factors have been reported especially clinically and immunologically active SLE, requiring non-active disease (clinically and immunologically) at the time of KT [10]. Clinically, recurrent LN presents with worsening proteinuria and graft function. Treatment of post-transplant relapse, including use of PEX, is practically the same as in LN in the general population [41].

Recurrent TMA after KT TMA has high recurrence rate, especially in those with complement factors H, I, B, and high titers of anti-complement factor H antibodies. Complement inhibition post-transplant is a reasonable approach to TMA relapse after KT [10]. Recurrent disease should be distinguished from de novo post-transplant TMA, commonly associated with the use of immunosuppressive agents, AbMR, viral infections. Treatment strategy in recurrent TMA is similar to the one in the general population and includes PEX, immunosuppression (IVIG,RTX), removal of triggering factors, and complement inhibitors (Eculizumab, Ravulizumab)—see Section PEX in TMA for details (Chap. 4) [3, 37].

Recurrent antiphospholipid syndrome (APS) after KT APS may relapse after KT or appear as de novo complication. APS should be clinically inactive at the time of KT; the importance of antiphospholipid Ab as risk factor for post-transplant APS relapse is unclear [10]. Generally, APS treatment consists of anticoagulation. However, in catastrophic APS (cAPS), defined as involvement of ≥3 organs/systems; rapid development of clinical symptoms (within 7 days); histological data for small vessel occlusion; and presence of antiphospholipid Ab, treatment with steroids, IVIG/RTX/Eculizumab, anticoagulation, and PEX are recommended as first-line treatment (see Section PEX in the Treatment of cAPS, Chap. 5) [42].

References

1. Philip D, PFH M. Minimal change nephrotic syndrome. In: Floege J, Johnson R, Feehaly J, editors. Comprehensive clinical nephrology. 4th ed. St. Louis: Elsevier Saunders; 2010. p. 218–27.
2. Rovin BH, Adler SG, Barratt J, Bridoux F, Burdge KA, Chan TM, et al. KDIGO 2021 clinical practice guideline for the management of glomerular diseases. Kidney Int. 2021;100(4S):S1–S276. https://doi.org/10.1016/j.kint.2021.05.021.
3. Connelly-Smith L, Alquist CR, Aqui NA, Hofmann JC, Klingel R, Onwuemene OA, et al. Guidelines on the use of therapeutic apheresis in clinical practice—evidence-based approach from the writing Committee of the American Society for apheresis: the ninth special issue. J Clin Apher. 2023;38(2):77–278. https://doi.org/10.1002/jca.22043.
4. Moret L, Ganea A, Dao M, Hummel A, Knebelman B, Subra JF, et al. Apheresis in adult with refractory idiopathic nephrotic syndrome on native kidneys. Kidney Int Rep. 2021;6(8):2134–43. https://doi.org/10.1016/j.ekir.2021.04.029.
5. Terada K, Mugishima K, Kawasaki S, Itagaki F, Yamada T, Sakai Y. Low-density lipoprotein apheresis in patients with acute kidney injury due to minimal change disease requiring acute renal replacement therapy. Int J Nephrol Renovasc Dis. 2020;13:157–62. https://doi.org/10.2147/IJNRD.S248610.
6. Brown EJ, Pollak MR, Barua M. Genetic testing for nephrotic syndrome and FSGS in the era of next-generation sequencing. Kidney Int. 2014;85(5):1030–8. https://doi.org/10.1038/ki.2014.48.
7. Shah L, Hooper DK, Okamura D, Wallace D, Moodalbail D, Gluck C, et al. LDL-apheresis-induced remission of focal segmental glomerulosclerosis recurrence in pediatric renal transplant recipients. Pediatr Nephrol. 2019;34(11):2343–50. https://doi.org/10.1007/s00467-019-04296-6.
8. Colucci M, Labbadia R, Vivarelli M, Camassei FD, Emma F, Dello Strologo L. Ofatumumab rescue treatment in post-transplant recurrence of focal segmental glomerulosclerosis. Pediatr Nephrol. 2020;35(2):341–5. https://doi.org/10.1007/s00467-019-04365-w.
9. Vallianou K, Marinaki S, Skalioti C, Lionaki S, Melexopoulou C, Boletis I, et al. Therapeutic options for recurrence of primary focal segmental glomerulonephritis (FSGS) in the renal allograft: single-center experience. J Clin Med. 2021;10(3):373. https://doi.org/10.3390/jcm10030373.
10. Chadban SJ, Ahn C, Axelrod DA, Foster BJ, Kasiske BL, Kher V, et al. KDIGO clinical practice guideline on the evaluation and management of candidates for kidney transplantation. Transplantation. 2020;104(4S1 Suppl 1):S11–S103. https://doi.org/10.1097/TP.0000000000003136.
11. Sethi S, Madden B. Mapping antigens of membranous nephropathy: almost there. Kidney Int. 2023;103(3):469–72. https://doi.org/10.1016/j.kint.2023.01.003.

12. Müller-Deile J, Schiffer L, Hiss M, Haller H, Schiffer M. A new rescue regimen with plasma exchange and rituximab in high-risk membranous glomerulonephritis. Eur J Clin Investig. 2015;45(12):1260–9. https://doi.org/10.1002/mco2.614.
13. Hamilton P, Kanigicherla D, Hanumapura P, Blaikie K, Ritchie J, Sinha S, et al. Peptide GAM immunoadsorption in anti-PLA2R positive autoimmune membranous nephropathy. The PRISM trial. J Clin Apher. 2022;37(1):40–53. https://doi.org/10.1002/jca.21949.
14. McAdoo SP, Pusey CD. Anti-glomerular basement membrane disease. Clin J Am Soc Nephrol. 2017;12(7):1162–72. https://doi.org/10.2215/CJN.01380217.
15. Ozkok A, Yildiz A. Hepatitis C virus associated glomerulopathies. World J Gastroenterol. 2014;20(24):7544–54. https://doi.org/10.3748/wjg.v20.i24.7544.
16. Iyengar A, Kamath N, Radhakrishnan J, Estebanez BT. Infection-related glomerulonephritis in children and adults. Semin Nephrol. 2023;43(5):151469. https://doi.org/10.1016/j.semnephrol.2023.151469.
17. KDIGO. Clinical practice guideline for the prevention, diagnosis, evaluation, and treatment of hepatitis C in chronic kidney disease. Kidney Int Suppl. 2018;8(3):91–165. https://doi.org/10.1016/j.kisu.2018.06.001.
18. Knoppova B, Reily C, Glenn King R, Julian BA, Novak J, Green TJ. Pathogenesis of Iga nephropathy: current understanding and implications for development of disease-specific treatment. J Clin Med. 2021;10(19):4501. https://doi.org/10.3390/jcm10194501.
19. Heineke MH, Ballering AV, Jamin A, Ben Mkaddem S, Monteiro RC, Van Egmond M. New insights in the pathogenesis of immunoglobulin A vasculitis (Henoch-Schönlein purpura). Autoimmun Rev. 2017;16(12):1246–53. https://doi.org/10.1016/j.autrev.2017.10.009.
20. Rovin BH, Barratt J, Cook HT, Noronha IL, Reich HN, Suzuki Y, et al. KDIGO 2025 clinical practice guideline for the management of immunoglobulin a nephropathy (IgAN) and immunoglobulin a vasculitis (IgAV). Kidney Int. 2025;108:S1–71. https://doi.org/10.1016/j.kint.2025.04.004.
21. Manohar S, Nasr SH, Leung N. Light chain cast nephropathy: practical considerations in the management of myeloma kidney—what we know and what the future may hold. Curr Hematol Malig Rep. 2018;13(3):220–6. https://doi.org/10.1007/s11899-018-0451-0.
22. Tarragón B, Ye N, Gallagher M, Sen S, Portolés JM, Wang AY. Effect of high cut-off dialysis for acute kidney injury secondary to cast nephropathy in patients with multiple myeloma: a systematic review and meta-analysis. Clin Kidney J. 2021;14(8):1894–900. https://doi.org/10.1093/ckj/sfaa220.
23. Kidney Disease: Improving Global Outcomes (KDIGO) Lupus Nephritis Work Group. KDIGO 2024 clinical practice guideline for the management of Lupus Nephritis. Kidney Int. 2024;105(1S):S1–S69. https://doi.org/10.1016/j.kint.2023.09.002.

24. Salvadori M, Tsalouchos A. Current protocols and outcomes of ABO-incompatible kidney transplantation. World J Transplant. 2020;10(7):191–205. https://doi.org/10.5500/wjt.v10.i7.191.
25. Ray DS, Thukral S. Outcome of ABO-incompatible living donor renal transplantations: a single-center experience from eastern India. Transplant Proc. 2016;48(8):2622–8. https://doi.org/10.1016/j.transproceed.2016.06.048.
26. Jha PK, Tiwari AK, Bansal SB, Sethi SK, Ahlawat R, Kher V. Cascade plasmapheresis as preconditioning regimen for ABO-incompatible renal transplantation: a single-center experience. Transfusion. 2016;56(4):956–61. https://doi.org/10.1111/trf.13427.
27. Tydén G, Kumlien G, Genberg H, Sandberg J, Lundgren T, Fehrman I. ABO incompatible kidney transplantations without splenectomy, using antigen-specific immunoadsorption and rituximab. Am J Transplant. 2005;5(1):145–8. https://doi.org/10.1111/j.1600-6143.2004.00653.x.
28. Malvezzi P, Jouve T, Noble J, Rostaing L. Desensitization in the setting of HLA-incompatible kidney transplant. Exp Clin Transplant. 2018;16(4):367–75. https://doi.org/10.6002/ect.2017.0355.
29. Kwon H, Kim JY, Kim DH, Ko Y, Choi JY, Shin S, et al. Effect of simultaneous presence of anti-blood group A/B and -HLA antibodies on clinical outcomes in kidney transplantation across positive crossmatch: a nationwide cohort study. Sci Rep. 2019;9(1):18229. https://doi.org/10.1038/s41598-019-54397-3.
30. Rostaing L, Congy N, Allal A, Esposito L, Sallusto F, Doumerc N, et al. Successful transplantation in ABO-and HLA-incompatible kidney-transplant patients. Transpl Int [Internet]. 2016;20(5):507–16. https://doi.org/10.1111/1744-9987.12408.
31. Loupy A, Haas M, Roufosse C, Naesens M, Adam B, Afrouzian M, et al. The Banff 2019 kidney meeting report (I): updates on and clarification of criteria for T cell– and antibody-mediated rejection. Am J Transplant. 2020;20(9):2318–31. https://doi.org/10.1111/ajt.15898.
32. Montgomery RA, Loupy A, Segev DL. Antibody-mediated rejection: new approaches in prevention and management. Am J Transplant. 2018;8(Suppl 3):3–17. https://doi.org/10.1111/ajt.14584.
33. Wiseman AC. Prophylaxis and treatment of kidney transplant rejection. In: Floege J, Johnson RJ, Floege J, editors. Comprehensive clinical nephrology. 4th ed. St Louis: Elsevier Saunders; 2010. p. 1166–76.
34. Coche S, Sprangers B, Van Laecke S, Weekers L, De Meyer V, Hellemans R, et al. Recurrence and outcome of anti–glomerular basement membrane glomerulonephritis after kidney transplantation. Kidney Int Rep. 2021;6(7):1888–94. https://doi.org/10.1016/j.ekir.2021.04.011.
35. Hullekes F, Uffing A, Verhoeff R, Seeger H, von Moos S, Mansur J, et al. Recurrence of membranous nephropathy after kidney transplantation: a multicenter retrospective cohort study. Am J Transplant. 2024;24(6):1016–26. https://doi.org/10.1016/j.ajt.2024.01.036.

36. Alasfar S, Carter-Monroe N, Rosenberg AZ, Montgomery RA, Alachkar N. Membranoproliferative glomerulonephritis recurrence after kidney transplantation: using the new classification. BMC Nephrol. 2016;17:7. https://doi.org/10.1186/s12882-015-0219-x.
37. Kidney Disease: Improving Global Outcomes (KDIGO) Transplant Work Group. KDIGO clinical practice guideline for the care of kidney transplant recipients. Am J Transplant. 2009;9(Suppl 3):S1–155. https://doi.org/10.1111/j.1600-6143.2009.02834.x.
38. Floege J, Jayne DRW, Sanders JSF, Tesar V, Rovin BH. KDIGO 2024 clinical practice guideline for the management of antineutrophil cytoplasmic antibody (ANCA)–associated vasculitis. Kidney Int. 2024;105(3S):S71–S116. https://doi.org/10.1016/j.kint.2023.10.008.
39. Nyberg G, Åkesson P, Nordén G, Wieslander J. Systemic vasculitis in a kidney transplant population. Transplantation. 1997;63(9):1273–7. https://doi.org/10.1097/00007890-199705150-00014.
40. Pattanaik D, Green J, Talwar M, Molnar M. Relapse and outcome of lupus nephritis after renal transplantation in the modern immunosuppressive era. Cureus. 2022;14(1):e20863. https://doi.org/10.7759/cureus.20863.
41. Jiang K, Pan Y, Pu D, Shi L, Xu X, Bai M, et al. Kidney transplantation in lupus nephritis: a comprehensive review of challenges and strategies. BMC Surg. 2025;25:112. https://doi.org/10.1186/s12893-025-02832-w.
42. Ambati A, Knight JS, Zuo Y. Antiphospholipid syndrome management: a 2023 update and practical algorithm-based approach. Curr Opin Rheumatol. 2023;35(3):149–60. https://doi.org/10.1097/BOR.0000000000000932.

Indications for PEX: Hematology

4

Abstract

The pathogenesis of a wide range of hematological diseases is based on the presence of autoantibodies or circulating immune complexes. Therefore, PEX can play a pivotal role in their therapy (e.g., thrombotic thrombocytopenic purpura, TTP). This chapter will discuss also the conservative treatment in other hematological issues that have become the major treatment option and in which the benefit from PEX is inconclusive (e.g., complement-mediated thrombotic microangiopathy, cmTMA). Additionally, less frequently used apheresis techniques will be reviewed (erythrocytapheresis, RBC exchange, leukocytapheresis, thrombocytapheresis) and their effectiveness in certain hematological conditions.

Keywords

Thrombotic microangiopathy (TMA) · Complement-mediated TMA · Thrombotic thrombocytopenic purpura · Hyperviscosity syndrome · ADAMTS13

J. J. Filipov, *Therapeutic Plasma Exchange*, In Clinical Practice, https://doi.org/10.1007/978-3-032-17275-4_4

Thrombotic Microangiopathies (TMAs)

TMAs are a wide range of conditions, histologically presenting with endothelial damage, formation of microvascular thrombi, and intimal artery edema. As the kidneys are the most common site of damage, renal involvement is characterized also by double contouring of GBM, mesangiolysis, and endotheliosis. Additionally, fragmented RBCs are pathognomonic for TMA. TMAs are generally recognized for the three major laboratory and clinical findings [1]:

- Low platelet count (below 100×10^9/l)
- Microangiopathic hemolytic anemia—Hb lower than 100 g/L, elevated lactate dehydrogenase (LDH), undetectable haptoglobulin, schistocytes on blood smear
- Organ involvement—kidneys, central nervous system (CNS), heart

TMAs have diverse etiology, leading to excessive thrombi formation, ischemic organ injury and mechanical fragmentation of RBC as they flow through the pathologically changed microvasculature [2]. PEX plays a different role in the treatment of the various TMA forms—it is first-line treatment in TTP, whereas in cmTMA its benefit is unclear. However, once TMA is suspected, PEX should be initiated, until TMA subtype is diagnosed.

Infection-Associated TMA (iaTMA)

Definition Infection-associated TMA is a condition, associated with colitis, hemolytic anemia, low PLT count, and usually kidney involvement, though other organs can also be affected (e.g., CNS). The disease affects predominantly children and accounts for up to 90% of all TMAs [3]. Shiga-like toxin producing strains of *Escherichia coli* (St-EC) are the most common etiology of iaTMA; other infectious agents (*Streptococcus pneumoniae*, viruses) can also trigger cmTMA.

Pathogenesis Shiga toxins are reabsorbed by globotriaosylceramide and the complex is deposited in endothelial cells, causing cellular damage and microvascular thrombi formation. Infection-associated TMA can present as secondary form of cmTMA too.

Clinical presentation Bloody diarrhea is the initial symptom; full-blown iaTMA is developed several days later. Additionally, vomiting, abdominal pain, fever and CNS involvement may be detected [4]. In other iaTMAs, the condition may present with sepsis and meningitis (*S. pneumoniae*).

Treatment Supportive treatment is generally recommended. Volume resuscitation should be performed; the use of antibiotics in iaTMA, caused by St-EC demonstrated poorer outcomes. Approximately 50% of the cases may require renal replacement treatment [3]. In iaTMA caused by other infections (e.g., *S. pneumoniae*), antibiotics are required.

PEX in the treatment of iaTMA Therapeutic apheresis is not the pivotal treatment in St-EC TMA, as its effectiveness is unclear. However, it may prove beneficial in cases with severe neurological involvement [5]. The following PEX characteristics have been suggested in St-EC TMA [6].

- Treatment volume per PEX: 1–1.5 EPV
- Interval between PEX procedures: 24 h
- Substitution fluid: FFP
- End of treatment: resolution of symptoms

Other iaTMA, presenting with cmTMA, similar PEX approach is suggested. However, *S. pneumoniae* exposes the Thomsen-Friedenreich (T-) antigen on the cell surface; PEX with FFP substitution may transfer anti-T-antibodies in the patient, which may cause antigen-antibody reaction and polyagglutination. Therefore, albumin substitution should be performed in these cases.

Complement-Mediated TMA (cmTMA)

Definition Complement-mediated TMA is a condition, presenting with low platelet count, hemolytic anemia, and organ damage (e.g., kidneys, heart, CNS), due to over-activation of the alternative pathway of the complement system (APCS). The disease is caused by inherited or acquired defects in the regulation of the complement system, though cmTMA can occur after infections, which are regarded as triggers of the disease [7].

Pathogenesis The APCS is activated via cascade activation of C3 and factor B, which leads to the formation of the complex C3bBb, which acts as C3 convertase and further potentiates the activation. Finally, C5 is activated; subsequently forming C5b-9 complex, which causes cell lysis. Inhibitors of the APCS are present—factor H, factor I, and membrane cofactor protein (MCP, CD46) [8]. The pathogenesis of cmTMA is based on genetic mutations, leading to dysregulation of regulatory proteins of APCS, causing over-activation and thrombi formation. A majority of these mutations lead to suppressed inhibitory regulators, especially factor H mutations. Autoantibodies can also suppress APCS inhibition (e.g., factor H autoantibodies) [9]. Genetic mutations of APCS activators (C3 and factor B) account for 40% of cmTMA cases. In the pathogenesis of secondary infection-associated cmTMA are involved the formation of antibodies, compromising Factor H inhibition, or neuraminidase activity (*S. pneumoniae,* Influenza A virus), which removes sialic acid from cell surface, making blood cells more vulnerable to APCS [7].

Clinical presentation The disease affects all genders and ages. Clinically, cmTMA presents with low platelet count, microangiopathic hemolytic anemia, schistocytes on blood smear, and AKI; additionally, hepatic and pancreatic involvement can be diagnosed. Rarely, CNS involvement is present (headache, seizures, and coma)—the finding is more typical for TTP. Immunology may demonstrate low C3, normal C4, normal CH50, low AP50, and normal ADAMTS13 activity (>10%); shiga toxin testing should be performed too [10].

Treatment The use of anti-C5 monoclonal antibodies, blocking C5 activation (Eculizumab, Ravulizumab) has improved significantly the outcomes of cmTMA. Additionally, other immunosuppressive agents can be used (steroids, RTX, cyclophosphamide) [10].

PEX in the treatment of cmTMA PEX should be initiated in all cases with suspected TMA, until TTP is excluded. Once TTP is ruled out, anti-C5 inhibition is recommended. Previously a key treatment option, currently PEX is not recommended in cmTMA as its effectiveness is unclear; Eculizumab/Ravulizumab proved to be effective therapies for achieving remission and for long-term treatment, including prevention of relapse after kidney transplantation [11]. However, PEX should be initiated until Eculizumab/Ravulizumab is available. The procedure is first line of treatment only in the presence of anti-Factor H antibodies (ASFA category 1) along with immunosuppressive agents (steroids, RTX, cyclophophamide).

- Treatment volume per PEX: 1–1.5 EPV.
- Interval between PEX procedures: 24 h.
- Substitution fluid: FFP or FFP/albumin.
- End of treatment: resolution of symptoms; individualized approach is needed [6].

Coagulation-Mediated TMAs

Definition Coagulation-mediated TMAs are rare conditions, associated with genetic mutations of several coagulation factors—diacylglycerol kinase-ε (DGKE), plasminogen, and thrombomodulin (TMD). The mutations present with the typical symptoms and findings for TMA; kidneys are affected predominantly by the disease.

Pathogenesis Genetic mutations in DGKE, plasminogen, or THBD cause defective activation of proteinase C (DGKE mutations), decreased fibrin degradation (plasminogen mutations), and impaired anticoagulation of thrombin and factor H (TMD), resulting in increased microthrombi formation [12].

Clinical presentation Except for the typical TMA symptoms, proteinuria, hematuria, hypertension, and CKD progression are present. DGKE mutations present clinically in newborns.

Treatment, including PEX Generally, supportive measures are suggested, as no specific treatment demonstrated clear benefit, including plasma infusions and C5 inhibition [13]. The data for PEX in coagulation-mediated TMA are scarce; therefore, the strategy for cmTMA is suggested, though the benefit is uncertain [6].

- Treatment volume per PEX: 1–1.5 EPV.
- Interval between PEX procedures: 24 h.
- Substitution fluid: FFP.
- End of treatment: no standard therapeutic plan exists, therapy is modified according the clinical and laboratory findings.

Thrombotic Thrombocytopenic Purpura (TTP)

Definition TTP is a life-threatening form of TMA, associated with very low to missing activity of ADAMTS13 (lower than 10%). Sometimes referred as ADAMTS13 variant TMA, the condition presents with the typical laboratory findings for TMA and various symptoms of organ damage, most typically cardiac, neurological, and renal [14, 15].

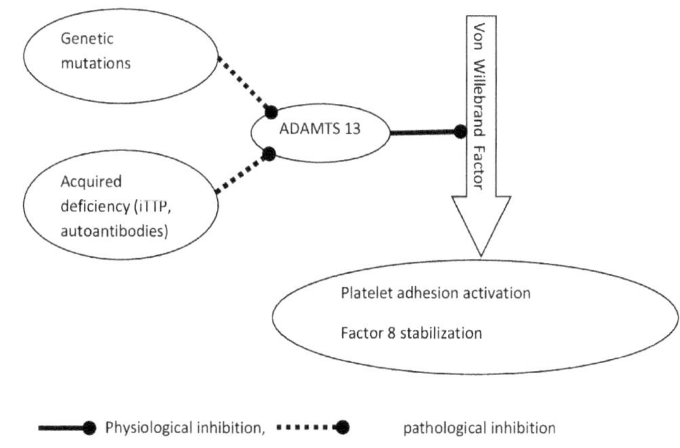

Fig. 4.1 Pathogenesis and pathophysiology of ADAMTS 13 deficiency in TTP

Pathogenesis ADAMTS 13 is a protease that cleaves von Willebrand factor (vWF), thus reducing its pro-thrombotic activity. In TTP, a low ADAMTS 13 activity (<10%) is present, inhibiting vWF function, causing extreme thrombosis. The condition can be linked to genetic mutations; however, acquired forms are more common and are caused by anti-ADAMTS 13 autoantibodies. Autoantibody-mediated TTP can be idiopathic or secondary to SLE, HIV infection, cancer [16]. Figure 4.1 demonstrates schematically the pathogenesis of ADAMTS 13 deficiency in TTP.

Clinical presentation Hemolytic anemia and thrombocytopenia (presenting with bleeding diathesis, petechiae) are the typical for TTP. End-organ damage is present too: CNS involvement (typical for TTP, may include seizures, headache, aphasia, dysarthria, and coma); cardiac symptoms (chest pain, myocardial infarction, cardiac arrest); renal involvement (usually less expressed, presenting with proteinuria, hematuria, AKI not characteristic); and intestinal symptoms (abdominal pain). The most important laboratory findings are the presence of schistocytes on blood smear, hemolysis, low PLT count (below 30×10^9/L), and low ADAMTS 13 activity (below 10%) [14, 16]. Remission is achieved when ADAMTS 13 activity is above 40%; a relapse is defined as ADAMATS 13 activity <20% after achieved remission [17].

Treatment. Role of PEX PEX plays a pivotal role in the therapy of TTP and is a first-line treatment of the condition (ASFA category 1). PEX removes pathogenic ADAMTS 13 autoantibodies and vWF multimers, and corrects enzyme deficiency by substituting with normal FFP. PEX should be coupled with immunosuppression (steroids, ≥1 mg/kg daily), Rituximab should be considered in the first acute TTP episode [18]. A novel agent Caplacizumab was introduced in the treatment of TTP recently. The medication targets the A1 domain of von Willebrand factor, preventing interaction with the platelet glycoprotein Ib-IX-V receptor and the development of thrombosis and demonstrated better outcomes, compared to PEX + steroids only. Plasma infusions are inferior to PEX and should be performed only in cases, in which PEX is not readily available, until the patient is transferred to institution, performing PEX [14].

- Treatment volume per PEX: 1.0–1.5 EPV.
- Interval between PEX procedures: 24 h.
- Substitution: FFP or FFP + albumin, or solvent/detergent-treated (S/D) plasma (lower risk for infection) [14].
- End of treatment: PEX to continue until normal PLT count for at least 2 consecutive days has been achieved [19]. Longer treatment with PEX at longer intervals have been tried, but without significant impact on TTP relapse rates [6].

Transplantation-Associated TMA (TA-TMA)

Definition TA-TMA is a condition characterized by hemolytic anemia, thrombocytopenia, and end-organ damage (kidneys,

CNS, heart) that occurs after successful solid organ transplantation (SOT) or hematopoietic stem cell transplantation (HSCT). TA-TMA can occur de novo or recur after organ transplantation (especially KT). Various etiological factors have been described for de novo TA-TMA: immunosuppressive medications (calcineurin inhibitors, CNI; mammalian target of Rapamycin inhibitors, mTORi), AbMR, infections [e.g., cytomegalovirus (CMV) infection], reperfusion injury, and deceased donation (especially KT) [20, 21]. Recurrent TMA post-transplant is associated with cmTMA and is based on genetic mutations in the regulators of APCS, most commonly Factor H mutations [22].

Pathogenesis TA-TMA pathogenesis is still not well defined. However, endothelial damage due to CNI, longer warm ischemia time, and AbMR may play a role in triggering TA post-transplant. A multiple hit theory in HSCT patients may explain post-transplant over-activation of complement system-predisposed individuals—first hit, endothelial damage—second hit, medications/infections/antibodies—the third hit [23]. TA-TMA is mostly complement mediated; ADAMTS 13 deficiency is unusual [24].

Clinical presentation The typical TMA symptoms and laboratory findings are present—hemolytic anemia, low PLT count, schistocytes on blood smear; end-organ damage is also present—CNS, renal involvement (proteinuria, decreased graft function), cardiac and pulmonary involvement, and gastrointestinal bleeding. It should be noted, that TA-TMA may present without thrombocytopenia and hemolysis in up to 30% of the cases; renal involvement is present in these situations, presenting with severe hypertension in younger patients and pathognomonic changes on graft biopsy [22]. Other laboratory findings include normal ADAMTS 13 activity, elevated soluble C5b-9, presence of anti-Factor H antibodies, elevated LDH, low haptoglobulin, and presence of donor-specific HLA antibodies are detected. In the setting of primary TMA prior to transplantation, genetic testing should be performed to exclude mutations.

Treatment Generally, no universal approach to TA-TMA exists. Causative agents (infections, AbMR) should be treated, as well as withdrawal of medications that may trigger TMA (CNI, mTORi). Additionally, treatment with Eculizumab was used with success in in TA-TMA in patients with genetic mutations, though chronic treatment may be needed [22].

Prevention of TA-TMA may include PEX + steroids + RTX regimen in the presence of Factor H autoantibodies in order to reduce Ab titer prior to transplantation. Chronic use of Eculisumab/Ravulizumab can also be considered in Factor H/factor I mutations, as well as combined kidney/liver transplantation [22].

PEX in the treatment of TA-TMA The benefit from PEX in TA-TMA is uncertain and its use is linked to adverse events and partial remissions, followed by disease relapses, both for SOT and HCPT (ASFA category 3). However, PEX may have more pronounced benefit in the presence of autoantibodies (e.g., anti-Factor H). Generally, the treatment regimen for TTP is applied, until improvement in laboratory and clinical symptoms is achieved; immunosuppressive protocols consist of steroids/RTX/Eculizumab [6].

- Treatment volume per PEX: 1.0–1.5 EPV.
- Interval between PEX procedures: 24 h.
- Substitution: FFP or FFP + albumin.
- End of treatment: until clinical and laboratory improvement is established.

Secondary TMA: Pregnancy-Associated TMA

Definition Pregnancy-associated TMA (pTMA) is a heterogeneous group of TMAs with microvascular thrombi formation. The major subtypes are as follows [1]:

1. Pre-eclampsia (PE) and hemolysis, elevated liver enzymes, low platelet count (HELLP) syndrome, usually developing after the 20th gestational week
2. TTP—occurring throughout all trimesters, with end-organ damage (predominantly CNS, milder kidney damage, heart)
3. cmTMA—occurring throughout all trimesters, may present after delivery, milder CNS involvement, more expressed kidney disease
4. APS-TMA, associated with Antiphospholipid syndrome (APS), due to persistent antiphospholipid antibodies, causing microvascular thrombosis in various organs

Pathogenesis

1. The pathogenesis of PE/HELLP syndrome is not fully clarified. However, abnormal placentation and impaired immune maternal-fetal tolerance were suggested as possible mechanisms. Additionally, impaired balance in complement system may lead to its over-activation, causing fetal and maternal symptoms. Finally, impaired balance between factors, causing vasoconstriction and endothelial damage (e.g., soluble fms-like tyrosine kinase 1, sFlt-1), and proangiogenic molecules (placental growth factor, PlGF) may trigger the complement system [25].
2. In pregnancy-associated TTP, a low ADAMTS 13 activity is detected. A possible explanation for decreased ADAMTS 13 activity is pregnancy-associated increase in vWF synthesis, which is an additional stress on ADAMTS 13 enzyme due to its consumption [26]. In the presence of genetic mutations and relatively low enzyme activity, the physiological stress in pregnancy provokes clinically significant enzyme deficiency.
3. The pathogenesis of cmTMA is based on over-activation of APCS (see section "Complement-Mediated TMA (cmTMA"). In pregnancy, a rise in regulators of complement activation is present to ensure placental protection. Post-partum decrease in complement inhibitors (MCP, CD59) occurs, which may trig-

ger cmTMA. Additionally, imbalance in pro-angiogenic and vasoconstrictor molecules may activate APCS [25].

4. The pathogenesis of APS-associated pTMA consists of multi-hit model: first hit is the presence of antiphospholipid antibodies, whereas the second hit includes the hormonal changes, occurring during pregnancy [27]. As a result inflammatory state is present, activating neutrophils, monocytes, leading to cell membrane disruption and complement activation.

Clinical presentation

1. PE/HELLP syndrome—presentation after 20th week of pregnancy; HELLP syndrome is the worst clinical presentation of PE. PE presents with gestational hypertension, proteinuria, and acute kidney injury; in addition, low PLT count, hemolysis (elevated LDH, low haptoglobulin), elevated liver enzymes may appear, contributing to the diagnosis HELLP syndrome. In eclampsia, the findings for PE are complicated with neurological symptoms—headache, blindness, abnormal mental status, and stroke. PE and/or HELLP syndrome and/or neurological symptoms is regarded as severe form of PE (PE-SF). Elevated sFlt-1/PlGF ratio is not enough to diagnose PE-SF [1].
2. Pregnancy-associated TTP may develop in any trimester, though it occurs more often in the third trimester and after delivery. TTP is the more frequent TMA during the first trimester. Clinically, pregnancy-associated TTP is similar to TTP in the general population. ADAMTS 13 activity is low (<10%). A testing for ant-ADAMTS 13 antibodies can be performed to differentiate immune TTP from congenital TTP.
3. Complement-mediated TMA in pregnancy usually occurs post-partum, within 3 months after delivery, though it can present at any trimester of pregnancy [1]. Clinically it presents with similar features and laboratory for cmTMA in the general population. Renal damage is usually more expressed than in TTP. Immunological testing may demonstrate low C3, normal

C4, normal CH50, low AP50, and normal ADAMTS13 activity (>10%).

4. APS-associated TMA in pregnancy presents with three distinct subtypes—thrombotic APS (presenting with arterial/venous thrombosis and micro-thrombi in different organs); obstetric (presenting with PE, recurrent fetal loss, premature birth); and catastrophic APS (multiorgan failure—kidneys, CNS, skin, etc., developing within a short period of time). A typical finding is the presence of antiphospholipid antibodies (lupus anticoagulant, anti-cardiolipin, and anti-b2GPI antibodies).

Treatment. Role of PEX In all types of pTMA prompt delivery is recommended, as it will be sufficient to treat the condition (PE/HELLP) or will enhance achieving remission (TTP, cmTMA) [1].

1. In PE/HELLP, delivery is the pivotal treatment. Symptoms for PE-SF should resolve within 72 h. In cases of persistent symptoms more than 72 h, other pTMAs should be considered (TTP, cmTMA) and PEX should be initiated as per TTP schedule—see section "Thrombotic Thrombocytopenic Purpura (TTP)". Earlier start of PEX may be indicated if life-threatening neurological and cardiac manifestations are present, as well as severe thrombocytopenia (PLT <30 × 10^9/L) [1]. Currently the benefit of PEX in HELLP syndrome is unclear (ASFA category 3); however, PEX prior to delivery is contraindicated (ASFA category 4), as it will postpone delivery, which is the treatment of choice [28].
2. In pregnancy-associated TTP, PEX should be initiated as per TTP protocol in the general population—see section "Thrombotic Thrombocytopenic Purpura (TTP)". In pregnant TTP cases, delivery can be postponed and performed if PEX has no effect on clinical and laboratory findings [1]. PEX should be coupled with immunosuppression (steroids, Azathiorpine, CNI); RTX should be used with caution as the molecule may cross the placenta and may cause fetal malfor-

mations [29]. First episodes of pregnancy associated genetic TTP and immune TTP are treated similarly with PEX and immunosuppression. In patients with a known genetic mutation of ADAMTS 13, prevention with FFP infusions is recommended, as TTP will relapse during pregnancy. FFP infusion starting from 10 mL/kg to 15 mL/kg plasma every 10–21 days is usually performed; doses can be increased in the second and third trimesters [30]. The risk for relapse of iTTP in next pregnancy is unknown. In these cases, ADAMTS 13 follow-up should be performed throughout the pregnancy, and treatment should be started at ADAMTS 13 below 20%. Initially steroids and Azathiorpine can be initiated, but in severe ADAMTS 13 activity reduction PEX should be started [31].

3. Complement-mediated TMA—PEX is started initially until TTP is excluded. Once cmTMA is diagnosed, anti-C5 treatment (Eculizumab/Ravulizumab) should be initiated. Larger doses and more frequent application of the medication may be needed due to increased C5 production and larger volume of distribution in pregnancy [1].
4. Pregnancy-associated APS-TMA—treatment is based on anticoagulation with low molecular weight heparins and Aspirin. However, in CAPS aggressive treatment with PEX, immunosuppressive agents (steroids, IVIG, RTX, Eculizumab) is needed. PEX is performed daily for 3–5 days, treatment volume—1-1.5 EPV, until symptoms resolve—see Section PEX in CAPS, Chap. 5 of this book.

Secondary TMA: Drugs

Definition Certain medications can cause TMA, presenting clinically with either TTP or cmTMA-associated symptoms. TMA is most commonly detected in CNI, mTOR inhibitors, Clopidugrel, hormonal preparations (estrogen/progesterone), gemcitabine, quinine use, but other medications (e.g., mytomycin, vincristin) were also reported to cause drug induced TMA (diTMA) [32].

Pathogenesis Various mechanisms have been suggested for diTMA. However, two principal mechanisms were detected: immune-mediated injury (Quinine, Gemcitabine) and direct toxic effect (dose dependent, acute or chronic toxicity—e.g., CNI, Sirolimus, interferon alfa, interferon beta). The two pathways can cause endothelial damage, over-activation of the complement system, suppression of ADAMTS 13 activity, leading to microthrombi formation [33].

Clinical presentation The symptoms and laboratory findings from the spectrum of TTP or cmTMA may be present. The relationship between medication and TMA episode can be used for diagnosis, but may be difficult to establish. Specific tests (presence of antibodies against PLT) can be performed.

Treatment Medication withdrawal or dose reduction is recommended. Additionally, immunosuppression (steroids, RTX, Eculizumab, Cyclophosphamide) and dialysis removal can be applied.

PEX in diTMA PEX was effective in immune diTMA, associated with antibodies against ADAMTS 13 (ticlodipine—ASFA category 1) and the treatment follows the TTP protocol—see section "Thrombotic Thrombocytopenic Purpura (TTP)". In diTMA, caused by agents with direct toxic effect PEX has unclear benefit (Clopidigrel, Mitomycin—ASFA category 3). In limited number of situations, PEX is contraindicated (Quinine, Gemcitabine—ASFA category 4).

- Treatment volume per PEX: 1.0–1.5 EPV.
- Interval between PEX procedures: 24 h.

- Substitution: FFP or FFP + albumin or solvent/detergent-treated (S/D) plasma [14].
- End of treatment: PEX to continue until normal PLT count for at least 2 consecutive days has been achieved [19]. Longer treatment with PEX at longer intervals have been tried, but without significant impact on TTP relapse rates [6].

TMA in Autoimmune Disease

Definition TMA can be secondary to autoimmune disease (e.g., SLE), as disease autoantibodies can influence complement system activity and cause microthrombi formation. Secondary TMA can be detected in other conditions—APS, systemic sclerosis (scleroderma renal crisis) [34].

Pathogenesis Antibodies associated with the autoimmune disease can cause APCS over-activation, by influencing suppressor activity; rare cases with SLE-associated autoantibodies against ADAMTS 13, causing SLE-associated TTP were described too [35]. Pathogenic changes may present on genetic background.

Clinical presentation The symptoms of underlying disease, coupled with those of TMA, are present. The typical laboratory findings for TMA are detected (hemolytic anemia, thrombocytopenia, elevated LDH, low haptoglobulin, schistocytes). In these cases, a detailed evaluation of the TMA type and autoimmune disease activity is required (SLE/APS autoantibodies, ADAMTS 13 activity, C3/C4 testing, factor H/I antibodies, genetic testing).

Treatment. Role of PEX Generally, treatment of underlying disease should be initiated. In refractory cases, anti-C5 treatment can be initiated. PEX is indicated in refractory autoimmune disease, complicated with TMA [6]. In systemic sclerosis, longer PEX treatment may be required

- Treatment volume per PEX: 1.0–1.5 EPV.
- Interval between PEX procedures: 24 h.
- Substitution: FFP or FFP + albumin or solvent/detergent-treated (S/D) plasma.
- End of treatment: PEX to continue until resolution of symptoms and improvement in laboratory tests. In systemic sclerosis, longer PEX treatment may be required [6].

Secondary TMA: Malignancy

Definition Malignancy-associated TMA (mTMA) clinical presentation ranges from asymptomatic laboratory findings to cmTMA or TTP, and usually is due to the neoplasia itself or a complication of the therapy/superimposed infection [36].

Pathogenesis mTMA can be caused by malignancy itself and is typical of mucin-secreting and metastatic malignancies (most commonly gastrointestinal, breast, prostate, and lung cancers). Tumor cells can directly activate clotting factors; tumor bone marrow invasion can also cause endothelial injury, which in turn leads to production of vWF multimers. ADAMTS 13 activity may be decreased too, but it is usually normal or mildly reduced in mTMA [36, 37]. Second, mTMA can be caused by chemotherapy and immune therapies—the pathogenesis of diTMA is outlined in section "Secondary TMA: Drugs".

Clinical presentation mTMA should be distinguished from other TMAs and other malignancy-associated complications. Patients tend to be older, pulmonary symptoms are more frequent in mTMA; signs for active malignancy should be sought. ADAMTS 13 activity is not severely reduced unlike primary TTP. Symptoms usually have longer duration in mTMA [37].

Treatment. Role of PEX Currently no consensus on the treatment exists. Generally, if mTMA is caused by medication, the drug should be stopped. Immunosuppressive treatment has no clear benefit.

PEX failed to demonstrate clear benefit in mTMA [36]. However, it may be useful in TTP and low ADAMTS 13 activity; therefore, PEX may be initiated until ADAMTS 13 results are present. Malignancy diagnosis should be performed too [38]. In drug-related mTMA, PEX also failed to improve outcomes (see section "Secondary TMA: Drugs").

Hypergammaglobulinemia-Associated Hyperviscosity

Definition Hyperviscosity syndrome (HVS) is a condition, presenting with neurological and visual disturbances, as well as mucosal bleeding. It is an oncological emergency. HVS may be due to elevated RBC, WBC, and PLT count, but most commonly it is associated with hypergammaglobulinemia, especially associated with Waldenström's disease [39].

Pathogenesis Elevated serum immunoglobulin (Ig) levels cause increased viscosity of blood, thus reducing blood flow in small vessels and causing hypoperfusion and impaired PLT aggregation. Hyperglobulinemia-associated HVS is caused by multiple myeloma; polyclonal HVS is present in HIV infection, Sjögren's syndrome, and rheumatoid arthritis [6].

Clinical presentation HVS presents with neurological symptoms (headache, seizures, neuropathic pain, coma); visual symptoms include double or blurred vision, with typical finding of "sausage link" engorgement of retinal vessels on fundoscopy. In addition, mucosal or skin bleeding is present. Rarely, cardiopulmonary symptoms (valvular dysfunction, shortness of breath, heart failure) may be diagnosed. Laboratory findings include elevated Ig levels (IgM. IgG, IgA); blood viscosity, measured in centipoise (cp) usually exceeds 2.2 cp [40].

Treatment. Role of PEX Hypergammaglomulinemia-associated HVS is an oncological emergency. PEX is a pivotal method in its treatment (ASFA category 1), as it removes paraproteins and quickly reduces viscosity and improves rapidly symptoms. As PEX has no influence in the underlying disease, adequate chemotherapy should be initiated too. PEX is particularly effective in Waldenström's disease, as IgM has 80% intravascular localization. One to three PEX procedures are sufficient for the symptoms to resolve; however, maintenance PEX may be needed—one procedure every 1–4 weeks. Prophylactic use of PEX prior to RTX infusion in Waldenström's disease is also effective in avoiding transient HVS [6].

- Treatment volume per PEX: 1.0–1.5 EPV.
- Interval between PEX procedures: 24–48 h.
- Substitution: albumin or FFP.
- End of treatment: improvement in symptoms (1–3 PEX); prophylactic PEX prior to RTX infusion—target IgM level <4 g/dl.

Autoimmune Hemolytic Anemia (AHA)

Definition AHA is a group of disorders, caused by autoantibodies, triggering intravascular or extravascular hemolysis. There are two major types—warm AHA, associated with autoantibodies, causing hemolysis optimally at 37 °C and cold agglutinin disease (CAD, autoantibodies cause hemolysis at temperatures in the range of 0–5 °C). Warm AHA is idiopathic, but may be secondary to autoimmune disease, lymphoproliferative diseases, and infection. CAD has similar etiology for secondary forms [41].

Pathogenesis Two major mechanisms were established in AHA—activation of the complex C5b-9 (in intravascular hemolysis) and macrophage-phagocytic-mediated extravascular RBC destruction. However, more complicated mechanisms have been described, including impaired T- and B cell regulation, impaired lymphocyte apoptosis, and acquired changes in RBC membranes that may cause hemolysis [42].

Clinical presentation AHA presents with the typical symptoms for hemolytic anemia—elevated LDH, unconjugated bilirubin, low haptoglobulin, normocytic anemia with spherocytes, and reticulocytosis. Positive direct anti-globulin test (DAT) for IgG and C3d is characteristic for AHA, though the test may be negative in up to 10% of the cases. Differential diagnosis should include autoimmune diseases, malignancies, infections (HIV, CMV, varicella, Epstein-Barr infection) [42]. Severe AHA is diagnosed in Hb <80 g/l or the need for transfusions.

Treatment Generally, treatment of the underlying disease, avoidance of low temperatures (CAD), and use of immunosuppressive agents (steroids, RTX, bortezomib).

PEX in AHA PEX is used in severe AHA, unresponsive to steroids. It is used as bridging therapy until novel immunosuppression achieves disease control (ASFA category 3 for warm AHA, ASFA category 2 for CAD).

In CAD, warmer room temperature may be required during the procedure [6].

- Treatment volume per PEX: 1.0–1.5 EPV
- Interval between PEX procedures: 24–48 h
- Substitution: albumin
- End of treatment: clinical improvement

Cryoglobulinemia

Definition Cryoglobulinemia is a pathological condition characterized with the aggregation of immunoglobulins in low temperatures (cryoglobulins), which potentially regain their solubility after warmer temperature is applied. Cryoglobilinemia has three distinct subtypes:

1. Type 1: consists of monoclonal Ig (IgG, IgA, IgM), as is associated with multiple myeloma, Waldenström macroglobulinemia, chronic lymphocytic leukemia, as well as monoclonal gammopathies, such as monoclonal gammopathy of undetermined significance (MGUS), or monoclonal gammopathy of clinical significance (MGCS) [43].
2. Type 2: consists of polyclonal IgG plus monoclonal IgM with rheumatoid-factor activity; its etiology is associated with infections [HCV, hepatitis B (HBV), HIV], autoimmune diseases (SLE, Sjögren syndrome), and lymphoproliferative disorders.
3. Type 3: consists of polyclonal IgG and/or polyclonal IgM, caused by infections (HCV), autoimmune diseases.

Types 2 and 3 are classified as mixed type cryoglobulinemia, HCV is of particular importance for its development [44].

Pathogenesis Type 1 and types 2 and 3 have distinct pathogenesis and pathophysiology. Type 1 cryoglobulinemia arises from pathological B cell line, producing monoclonal Ig, which precipitates at low temperatures, causing microvascular obstruction and end-organ ischemia. In types 2 and 3, HCV infection is the leading etiology; HCV can induce B cell proliferation and activation, which in turn leads to Ig production. Initially causing polyclonal production, a persistent viral stimulation causes monoclonal Ig production with rheumatoid factor activity. Finally, cryoglobulin-associated immune complexes are formed, causing complement activation and small vessel vasculitis [43].

Clinical presentation Type 1 usually presents with signs of ischemia, skin lesions—livedo reticularis/skin necrosis. Types 2/3 may present with signs of small vessel vasculitis: peripheral polyneuropathy; palpable purpura, arthralgia, renal involvement—membranoproliferative glomerulonephritis and CNS involvement (stroke, coma). Advancing clinical picture, with involvement of CNS, gastrointestinal bleeding, and other life-threatening end-organ involvement is regarded as severe cryoglobulinemia. The diagnosis is made by detecting cryoglobulins; the cryocrit values are elevated (>0.5%). Additionally, low increased rheumatoid factor activity, C4, and CH50 are detected.

Treatment Generally, treatment of the underlying disease and immunosuppression (steroids, cyclophosphamide, RTX) are recommended. In cryoglobulinemia vasculitis, maintenance RTX treatment may be needed [45].

PEX in cryoglobulinemia PEX is a second-line treatment in cryoglobulinemia. It is indicated in severe forms with rapid renal involvement, life-threatening organ involvement, and hyperviscosity syndrome (cryocrit >10%) [44]. Other therapeutic apheresis techniques can be used too—DFPP and cryofiltration. Immunosuppression and treatment of underlying disease should be performed along with PEX/DFPP/cryofiltration; this treatment demonstrated excellent results in all types of cryoglobulinemia with renal involvement [46]. The following PEX schedule is suggested [6]:

- Treatment volume per PEX: 1.0–1.5 EPV.
- Interval between PEX procedures: ranges from 24 to 72 h, maintenance PEX may be required.
- Substitution: albumin.
- End of treatment: improvement in symptoms. Cryocrit should not be used to guide PEX treatment.

Hematopoietic Stem Cell Transplantation (HSCT)

AB0i HSCT

Definition and pathophysiology There are three types of AB0-incompatible allogenic HSCT—major AB0i HSCT, minor AB0i HSCT, and bidirectional (both major and minor incompatibility). In major AB0-incompatible HSCT, natural isoagglutinins in the recipient against the donors' A and/or B blood group antigens are present. They cause acute hemolysis of the RBCs present in infused hematopoietic progenitor cell (HPC) products—especially bone marrow HPC products—as well as prolonged RBC engraftment after HSCT. Additional complication may be pure red cell aplasia (PRCA).

In minor AB0 incompatible HSCT, donor isoagglutinins in HPC can cause hemolysis by reacting with A-/B antigens on host RBC membrane; however, clinically significant hemolysis is present only if the antibodies are in high titers or higher volume of plasma infused (>200 ml).

Finally, both major and minor AB0i HSCT may be present [47].

Though AB0 incompatibility is not regarded as a major obstacle to HSCT, it is associated with poorer post-transplant outcomes, compared to matched HSCT [48].

Clinical presentation AB0i-HSCT can cause hemolysis, delayed RBC engraftment, and PRCA.

Treatment and role of PEX Generally, pre-transplant RBC depletion of HPC; alternatively, reduction of isoagglutinin titers in recipients by using PEX is performed prior to major AB0i-HSCT. PEX can be performed post-transplant in cases of PRCA, but the benefit is unclear. In minor AB0i-HSCT a single RBC exchange to reduce donor-incompatible RBC can be applied [6].

Major AB0i-HSCT:

- Treatment volume per PEX: 1.0–1.5 EPV
- Interval between PEX procedures: 24 h
- Substitution: albumin or compatible for donor and recipient FFP
- End of treatment: target isoagglutinin titer <1:16

Minor AB0i-HSCT:

- Treatment volume for RBC exchange: 1–1.5 RBC volumes
- Number of RBC exchange: single procedure
- Substitution: RBC, blood group 0

HLA Desensitization in Allogenic HSCT

Definition The presence of donor-specific HLA antibodies (DSA-HLA Ab) prior to allogenic HSCT is associated with increased risk for graft failure. Different MFI cut-off values for DSA-HLA Ab for graft failure were reported, with MFI ranging from 2000 to 5000 [49].

Pathogenesis and clinical significance DSA-HLA Ab cause complement-mediated or Ab-dependent cell-mediated cytotoxicity of stem cells. Their presence is associated with poorer graft function, impaired engraftment, and higher risk for rejection [49].

Treatment. Role of PEX Ideally, donor selection, avoiding recipient incompatibility (HLA antigens, targeted by recipient's HLA antibodies) should be performed. If donor selection is impossible, desensitization protocols, based on PEX and immunosuppression (steroids, RTX, bortezomib, IVIG, tacrolimus and mycophenolate mofetil), as well as HLA matched hyperplatelet infusions can be applied. Desensitization protocols start 7–14 days prior to conditioning. Patients with low MFI (<3000) may not require desensitization [49]. PEX in HSCT HLA desensitization removes DSA-HLA Ab and is currently classified as ASFA category 3. Technically, the following PEX protocol is recommended [6, 49]:

- Treatment volume per PEX: 1.0 EPV.
- Interval between PEX procedures: 48 h.
- Substitution: albumin.
- End of treatment: until significant MFI reduction, suggestive of a negative flow cytometric crossmatch prior to HSCT is achieved.

Graft Versus Host Disease (GVHD)

Definition GVHD is a syndrome caused by immunologically active donor cells attack host tissues after HSCT. It represents with various clinical symptoms, most often engaging skin, mucosa, gastrointestinal tract, liver, and lungs. It has two forms, acute GVHD (aGVHD) and chronic GVHD (cGVHD); initially the two types were differentiated according to the time of presentation after HSCT, but current differentiation is based more on clinical presentation [50]. GVHD is associated with significant morbidity and mortality.

Pathogenesis ant pathophysiology Acute GVHD is initiated by host organ damage during conditioning regimen. This leads to activation and expansion of clonal T cells, which produce inflammatory cytokines and cause tissue damage. In the pathogenesis of cGVHD persistent of alloreactive donor T cells, activated recipient T cells and chronic inflammation have been described.

Clinical presentation Acute GVHD presents with the following clinical symptoms: skin lesions (e.g., maculopapular rash), cholestasis and/or acute hepatitis, gingivitis, diarrhea, vomiting, and lung involvement—bronchiolitis obliterans. Chronic GVHD presents with similar organ involvement, but demonstrating fibrotic changes: skin (depigmentation, sclerotic changes, poikilodermia, nail loss), mucosal involvement—xerostomia, hyperkeratotic plaques; esophageal strictures and stenosis, dry and painful eyes, ascites, and nephrotic syndrome. Some of the features between aGVHD and cGVHD may overlap [51].

Treatment A first-line treatment for GVHD grades II-IV is systemic immunosuppression (steroids, Alemtuzumab, Infliximab, mycophenolate preparations). In cGVHD, a similar approach is used in moderate to severe forms (steroids, CNI, mycophenolate, RTX) [50].

Therapeutic apheresis in GVHD Extracorporeal photopheresis (ECP) is suggested as second-line treatment in GVHD. The principles of ECP have been outlined in section "Leukocytapheresis" in Chap. 2 of this book. Two types of ECP are present—in-line ECP, in which UVA radiation occurs during the centrifugation of leukocytes and off-line ECP, in which WBC separation and UVA radiation occur in different devices, so the patient is disconnected from the separation device once WBC separation is accomplished. In-line ECP processes 1.5 L of blood, 2 procedures in 2 consecutive days are regarded as one cycle; in off-line ECP, larger blood volumes may be processed (3.5–10 L). Due to the higher volumes, a single procedure was found to be equivalent to one in-line ECP cycle in GVHD [52]. Generally, the procedure is well tolerated; however, major obstacles can be vascular access (peripheral access preferred) and low PLT count (PLT $<30 \times 10^9$/L) [50]. The following treatment schedules have been proposed [6, 52]:

Acute GVHD:

- Treatment schedule: 1 treatment cycle weekly until response occurs, then reduced to 1 cycle/14 days; up to 8 weeks of treatment. More intensive initial treatment of 2 cycles weekly can be initiated, especially in grade IV aGVHD and gastrointestinal involvement.

- End of treatment: improvement of symptoms and reduction of steroid doses are indicators for clinical response. However, abrupt cessation of ECP is rarely performed, as ECP should be performed at increased intervals, most commonly up to 8 weeks.

Chronic GVHD:

- Treatment schedule: 1 treatment cycle weekly or per 2 weeks up to 3 months, then reduced to 1 cycle/month. Intensive initial treatment has no benefit in cGVHD.
- End of treatment: depends on clinical response. If no benefit detected within 3 months, stop ECP.

Sickle Cell Disease (SCD)

Definition SCD is a hereditary disease characterized with the production of abnormal hemoglobin S (HbS), which causes crescent-like deformation of RBC. Abnormal RBCs have increased stiffness and reduce their ability to pass through smaller vessels. Abnormal RBCs have shorter life span and cause chronic hemolysis. Under certain conditions, RBCs cause vascular occlusion and acute symptoms such as end-organ ischemia.

Pathogenesis and pathophysiology The synthesis of pathologic HbS due to genetic mutation is the primary defect in SCD. Under certain conditions (stress, hypoxia, infection, dehydration, exposure to cold), HbS forms polymers, causing a change in the shape of RBC (sickle cells), which are rigid and easily undergo hemolysis. Sickle cells easily form aggregates, adhere to endothelium, thus blocking microvascular blood flow and causing tissue ischemia. Increased viscosity in SCD can further complicate microvascular event and worsens tissue ischemia [53].

Clinical picture Acute SCD presents with vaso-occlusive crises, which may present with episodes of pain in the extremities, acute chest syndrome (ACS), acute stroke, splenic sequestration, as well as long-term complications: chronic kidney disease, retinopathy, and avascular bone necrosis. Other chronic complications are chronic hemolysis, chronic pain, and pulmonary hypertension [54].

Treatment of SCD. Role of RBC exchange Disease-modifying therapies (Hydroxyurea, L-glutamine, crizanlizumab) have been used to control and prevent acute symptoms, as well as chronic RBC transfusions. In acute episodes, hydration, pain management, antibiotics, and oxygen supplementation should be performed. In SCD-associated stroke and ACS, RBC exchange is indicated; RBC exchange is first-line treatment in acute neurological symptoms (ASFA category 1). RBC exchange can be used also in acute episode prevention, especially in stroke prevention (ASFA category 1).

1. RBC exchange schedule of acute SCD [6, 54]:
    - Treatment volume: treatment volume should achieve target HbS below 30% and end hematocrit ≤33%; it can be calculated automatically. Fixed exchange of 1.5 RBC volume can also be applied.
    - Number of procedures: single RBC exchange.
    - Substitution fluid: leucocyte reduced RBC units, antigen matched.
    - Target: HbS <30%.
2. RBC exchange in chronic SCD.
    - Indication for chronic RBC exchange: stroke prevention (ASFA category 1), as well as in pregnancy and recurrent vascular occlusions [6].
    - Treatment volume: treatment volume should achieve target HbS below 30% and end hematocrit ≤33%; it can be calculated automatically. Lower HbS may be needed to keep HbS below 30% till the next procedure. Fixed exchange of 1.5 RBC volume can also be applied.

- Substitution fluid: see RBC exchange in acute SCD.
- Interval between RBC exchange—aiming at HbS <30%.

Erythrocytosis

Definition Erythrocytosis is defined as elevated RBC count above normal sex-related upper limits. Erythrocytosis can be classified as relative (due to dehydration) and absolute; as well as primary (due to autonomous RBC production, mainly due to polycythemia vera) and secondary (hypoxemia, local renal hypoxemia, erythropoietin-producing tumors, and drug related) [55].

Pathogenesis and pathophysiology Polycythemia vera (PV) is characterized with autonomous RBC production. Secondary erythrocytosis can be caused by generalized hypoxemia due to lung disease, right to left cardiopulmonary shunt, high altitude. Local renal ischemia (renal artery stenosis, autosomal polycystic kidney disease, hydronephrosis) also causes increased erythropoietin synthesis. Finally, erythropoietin-producing tumors (e.g., renal cell carcinoma) and medications (testosterone amd erythropoiesis stimulating agents) can cause secondary erythrocytosis. Elevated RBC count increases viscosity of blood, causing thromboses and symptoms similar to HVS (Section "Hypergammaglobulinemia-Associated Hyperviscosity").

Clinical presentation The two major types of erythrocytosis may be asymptomatic. Arterial and venous thromboses are a typical complication, in addition to vasomotor symptoms (headache, visual abnormalities) and erythromelalgia. Polycythemia vera can be diagnosed by detection of JAK2 mutations, bone marrow biopsy showing panmyelosis. Secondary etiology of elevated RBC should be meticulously searched.

Treatment. Role of therapeutic apheresis (erythrocytapheresis) In secondary forms, treatment of underlying disease is crucial, accompanied by acetyl salicylic acid prophylaxis. In PV, acetyl salicylic acid prophylaxis and phlebotomy are needed; cytoreductive treatment is required in high-risk PV.

Erythrocytapheresis and phlebotomy aim at hematocrit level <45%. Erythrocytapheresis is more effective than phlebotomy in correcting RBC count and in controlling symptoms. The principles of erythrocytapheresis have been described in section "Erythrocytapheresis" in Chap. 2 of this book. The procedure is effective in resolving the symptoms in PV (ASFA category 1) [6].

- Treatment volume: individually defined by TBV, initial and target hematocrit.
- Substitution fluid: albumin + saline.
- Interval between procedures; end of treatment: treatment schedule depends on the achieved target hematocrit; resolution of symptoms, as well as the effect of other disease specific therapies.

Thrombocytosis

Definition Thrombocytosiis is generally defined as PLT count >450 × 10^9/L. Thrombocytosis can be primary due to clonal proliferation [e.g., essential thrombocytosis (ET), PV, primary myelofibrosis]; reactive, due to infection, inflammation, tissue injury, and malignancy. Rarely spurious thrombocytosis is present, associated with cryoglobulinemia and circulating fragments from leukemic cells [56].

Pathogenesis and pathophysiology In primary thrombocytosis, clonal proliferation is associated with JAK2, CALR, and MPL somatic mutations. Reactive thrombocytosis is associated with the presence of pro-inflammatory cytokines in infection, inflammation, cancer, which influence thrombopoiesis.

Clinical presentation Increased PLT count in reactive thrombocytosis is rarely associated with thrombotic complications. They are more common in primary thrombocytosis. Microvascular thrombosis, engaging small vessels, usually presents with vasomotor symptoms, described in section "Erythrocytosis". Macrovascular thrombosis, involving larger arteries (CNS, coronary arteries) and veins (splanchnic veins) are also detected. Additionally, bleeding diathesis may be present due to functional abnormalities of clonal PLT and acquired von Willebrand syndrome [56]. General symptoms such as fever, sweating, and weight loss may be present too.

Treatment. Role of therapeutic apheresis (thrombocytapheresis) In reactive forms, treatment of underlying disease is indicated. In ET and PV, low-dose acetyl salicylic acid and cytoreductive therapy are recommended.

Thrombocytapheresis is described in section "Thrombocytapheresis" in Chap. 2 of this book. Currently it is used as bridging therapy in symptomatic thrombocytosis, until cytoreductive therapy effectively controls the disease. Its prophylactic use has unclear benefit in thrombocytosis. The following therapeutic schedule is recommended [6]:

- Treatment volume per session: 1.5–2.0 TBV.
- Substitution fluid: albumin + saline.
- Target of therapy. End of treatment: Target PLT count $<450 \times 10^9$/L. Treatment is to continue until underlying disease is effectively under control by cytoreductive therapy.

Hyperleukocytosis

Definition Hyperleukocytosis is defined as WBC count $>100 \times 10^9$/L and is associated with leukemia—acute myeloid leukemia (AML), but also acute lymphoblastic leukemia (ALL), chronic lymphocytic leukemia (CLL), and chronic myeloid leukemia (CML), especially in blast crisis.

Pathogenesis and pathophysiology High number of clonal cells causes increased blood viscosity, leading to leukostasis in small vessels and ischemia and tissue damage. Malignant cells have higher turnover, causing spontaneous or drug-induced tumor lysis syndrome (TLS); additionally, higher malignant cell turnover causes release of tissue factor, which activates factor IIV and leading to disseminated intravascular coagulopathy (DIC) [57].

Clinical presentation Leukostasis is associated with hyperviscosity and resemble the clinical findings described in ET and PV (Sections "Hypergammaglobulinemia-Associated Hyperviscosity", "Erythrocytosis", and "Thrombocytosis" of this chapter). Leukostasis is more common in AML due to the larger size of the clonal cells, compared to ALL and CLL. Additionally, manifestations of DIC (low platelet count, bleeding diathesis, low fibrinogen level) are present, as well as TLS (presenting with acute kidney injury).

Treatment. Role of therapeutic apheresis Generally, the treatment of hyperleukocytosis is cytoreductive treatment of the underlying disease. The apheresis method used is leukocytapheresis. The method is explained in detail in section "Leukocytapheresis" in Chap. 2. Unfortunately, leukocytapheresis has unclear benefit in the short-and long-term survival; currently its use is mainly limited to relieving leukostasis symptoms, until cytoreductive treatment effectively controls the disease [6, 58]. The following schedule is suggested:

- Treatment volume per session: 1.5–2.0 TBV.
- Interval between sessions: 24 h.
- Substitution fluid: saline + albumin, rarely FFP.
- Target of therapy. End of treatment: Target of treatment WBC $<50 \times 10^9$/L and resolution of symptoms.

References

1. Fakhouri F, Scully M, Provot F, Blasco M, Coppo P, Noris M, et al. Management of thrombotic microangiopathy in pregnancy and postpartum: report from an international working group. Blood. 2020;136(19):2103–17. https://doi.org/10.1182/blood.2020005221.
2. Genest DS, Patriquin CJ, Licht C, John R, Reich HN. Renal thrombotic microangiopathy: a review. Am J Kidney Dis. 2023;81(5):591–605. https://doi.org/10.1053/j.ajkd.2022.10.014.
3. Joseph A, Cointe A, Kurkdjian PM, Rafat C, Hertig A. Shiga toxin-associated hemolytic uremic syndrome: a narrative review. Toxins (Basel). 2020;12(2):67. https://doi.org/10.3390/toxins12020067.
4. McFarlane PA, Bitzan M, Broome C, Baran D, Garland J, Girard LP, et al. Making the correct diagnosis in thrombotic microangiopathy: a narrative review. Can J Kidney Health Dis. 2021;8:20543581211008707. https://doi.org/10.1177/20543581211008707.
5. Nathanson S, Kwon T, Elmaleh M, Charbit M, Launay EA, Harambat J, et al. Acute neurological involvement in diarrhea-associated hemolytic uremic syndrome. Clin J Am Soc Nephrol. 2010;5(7):1218–28. https://doi.org/10.2215/CJN.08921209.
6. Connelly-Smith L, Alquist CR, Aqui NA, Hofmann JC, Klingel R, Onwuemene OA, et al. Guidelines on the use of therapeutic apheresis in clinical practice – evidence-based approach from the writing Committee of the American Society for apheresis: the ninth special issue. J Clin Apher. 2023;38(2):77–278. https://doi.org/10.1002/jca.22043.
7. Sakari JT. HUS and atypical HUS. Blood. 2017;129(21):2847–56. https://doi.org/10.1182/blood-2016-11-709865.
8. Thompson GL, Kavanagh D. Diagnosis and treatment of thrombotic microangiopathy. Int J Lab Hematol. 2022;44(Suppl 1):101–13. https://doi.org/10.1111/ijlh.13954.
9. Dragon-Durey MA, Loirat C, Cloarec S, Macher MA, Blouin J, Nivet H, et al. Anti-factor H autoantibodies associated with atypical hemolytic uremic syndrome. J Am Soc Nephrol. 2005;16(2):555–63. https://doi.org/10.1681/ASN.2004050380.
10. Afshar-Kharghan V. Atypical hemolytic uremic syndrome. Hematology. 2016;2016(1):217–25. https://doi.org/10.1182/asheducation-2016.1.217.
11. Zuber J, Fakhouri F, Roumenina LT, Loirat C, Frémeaux-Bacchi V. Use of eculizumab for atypical haemolytic uraemic syndrome and C3 glomerulopathies. Nat Rev Nephrol. 2012;8(11):643–57. https://doi.org/10.1038/nrneph.2012.214.
12. Go RS, Winters JL, Leung N, Murray DL, Willrich MA, Abraham RS, et al. Thrombotic microangiopathy care pathway: a consensus statement for the Mayo Clinic complement alternative pathway-thrombotic micro-

angiopathy (CAP-TMA) disease-oriented group. Mayo Clin Proc. 2016;91(9):1189–211. https://doi.org/10.1016/j.mayocp.2016.05.015.

13. Epand RM, So V, Jennings W, Khadka B, Gupta RS, Lemaire M. Diacylglycerol kinase-ε: properties and biological roles. Front Cell Dev Biol. 2016;4:112. https://doi.org/10.3389/fcell.2016.00112.
14. Scully M, Rayment R, Clark A, Westwood JP, Cranfield T, Gooding R, et al. A British Society for Haematology guideline: diagnosis and management of thrombotic thrombocytopenic purpura and thrombotic microangiopathies. Br J Haematol. 2023;203(4):546–63. https://doi.org/10.1111/bjh.19026.
15. Aigner C, Schmidt A, Gaggl M, Sunder-Plassmann G. An updated classification of thrombotic microangiopathies and treatment of complement gene variant-mediated thrombotic microangiopathy. Clin Kidney J. 2019;12(3):333–7. https://doi.org/10.1093/ckj/sfz040.
16. Joly BS, Coppo P, Veyradier A. Thrombotic thrombocytopenic purpura. Blood. 2017;129(21):2836–46. https://doi.org/10.1182/blood-2016-10-709857.
17. Cuker A, Cataland SR, Coppo P, de la Rubia J, Friedman KD, George JN, et al. Redefining outcomes in immune TTP: an international working group consensus report. Blood. 2021;137(14):1855–61. https://doi.org/10.1182/blood.2020009150.
18. Zheng XL, Vesely SK, Cataland SR, Coppo P, Geldziler B, Iorio A, et al. ISTH guidelines for treatment of thrombotic thrombocytopenic purpura. J Thromb Haemost. 2020;18(10):2496–502. https://doi.org/10.1111/jth.15010.
19. Scully M, Cataland SR, Peyvandi F, Coppo P, Knöbl P, Kremer Hovinga JA, et al. Caplacizumab treatment for acquired thrombotic thrombocytopenic purpura. N Engl J Med. 2019;380(4):335–46. https://doi.org/10.1056/NEJMoa1806311.
20. Ávila A, Gavela E, Sancho A. Thrombotic microangiopathy after kidney transplantation: an underdiagnosed and potentially reversible entity. Front Med. 2021;8:642864. https://doi.org/10.3389/fmed.2021.642864.
21. Jodele S, Dandoy CE, Sabulski A, Koo J, Lane A, Myers KC, et al. Transplantation-associated thrombotic microangiopathy risk stratification: is there a window of opportunity to improve outcomes? Transplant Cell Ther. 2022;28(7):392.e1–9. https://doi.org/10.1016/j.jtct.2022.04.019.
22. Noris M, Remuzzi G. Thrombotic microangiopathy after kidney transplantation. Am J Transplant. 2010;10(7):1517–23. https://doi.org/10.1111/j.1600-6143.2010.03156.x.
23. Dvorak CC, Higham C, Shimano KA. Transplant-associated thrombotic microangiopathy in pediatric hematopoietic cell transplant recipients: a practical approach to diagnosis and management. Front Pediatr. 2019;7:133. https://doi.org/10.3389/fped.2019.00133.

24. Young JA, Pallas CR, Knovich MA. Transplant-associated thrombotic microangiopathy: theoretical considerations and a practical approach to an unrefined diagnosis. Bone Marrow Transplant. 2021;56(8):1805–17. https://doi.org/10.1038/s41409-021-01283-0.
25. Urra M, Lyons S, Teodosiu CG, Burwick R, Java A. Thrombotic microangiopathy in pregnancy: current understanding and management strategies. Kidney Int Rep [Internet]. 2024;9:2353–71. https://doi.org/10.1016/j.ekir.2024.05.016.
26. Mannucci PO, Canciani MT, Forza I, Lussana F, Lattuada A, Rossi E. Changes in health and disease of the metalloprotease that cleaves von Willebrand factor. Blood. 2001;98(9):2730–5. https://doi.org/10.1182/blood.v98.9.2730.
27. Urbanus RT, Siegerink B, Roest M, Rosendaal FR, de Groot PG, Algra A. Antiphospholipid antibodies and risk of myocardial infarction and ischaemic stroke in young women in the RATIO study: a case-control study. Lancet Neurol. 2009;8:998–1005. https://doi.org/10.1016/S1474-4422(09)70239-X.
28. Padmanabhan A, Connelly-Smith L, Aqui N, Balogun RA, Klingel R, Meyer E, et al. Guidelines on the use of therapeutic apheresis in clinical practice - evidence-based approach from the writing Committee of the American Society for apheresis: the eighth special issue. J Clin Apher. 2019;34:171–354. https://doi.org/10.1002/jca.21705.
29. Chakravarty EF, Murray ER, Kelman A, Farmer P. Pregnancy outcomes after maternal exposure to rituximab. Blood. 2011;117(5):1499–506. https://doi.org/10.1182/blood-2010-07-295444.
30. Ferrari B, Peyvandi F. How I treat thrombotic thrombocytopenic purpura in pregnancy. Blood. 2020;136(19):2125–32. https://doi.org/10.1182/blood.2019000962.
31. Scully M, Neave L. Etiology and outcomes: thrombotic microangiopathies in pregnancy. Res Pract Thromb Haemost [Internet]. 2023;7:100084. https://doi.org/10.1016/j.rpth.2023.100084.
32. Al-Nouri ZL, Reese JA, Terrell DR, Vesely SK, George JN. Drug-induced thrombotic microangiopathy: a systematic review of published reports. Blood. 2015;125:616–8. https://doi.org/10.1182/blood-2014-11-611335.
33. Mazzierli T, Allegretta F, Maffini E, Allinovi M. Drug-induced thrombotic microangiopathy: an updated review of causative drugs, pathophysiology, and management. Front Pharmacol. 2023;13:1–15. https://doi.org/10.3389/fphar.2022.1088031.
34. Java A, Kim AHJ. The role of complement in autoimmune disease-associated thrombotic microangiopathy and the potential for therapeutics. J Rheumatol. 2023;50:730–40. https://doi.org/10.3899/jrheum.220752.
35. Takagi Y, Kobayashi Y, Hirakata A, Takei M, Ogasawara S, Yajima C, et al. Systemic lupus erythematosus presenting with thrombotic thrombocytopenic purpura at onset: a case report. Front Pediatr. 2022;10:931669. https://doi.org/10.3389/fped.2022.931669.

36. Font C, de Herreros MG, Tsoukalas N, Brito-Dellan N, Espósito F, Escalante C, et al. Thrombotic microangiopathy (TMA) in adult patients with solid tumors: a challenging complication in the era of emerging anticancer therapies. Support Care Cancer. 2022;30(10):8599–609. https://doi.org/10.1007/s00520-022-06935-5.
37. Babu KG, Bhat GR. Cancer-associated thrombotic microangiopathy. Ecancermedicalscience. 2016;10:1–11. https://doi.org/10.3332/ecancer.2016.649.
38. Winters JL. Plasma exchange in thrombotic microangiopathies (TMAs) other than thrombotic thrombocytopenic purpura (TTP). Hematology. 2017;1:632–8. https://doi.org/10.1182/asheducation-2017.1.632.
39. Espinosa-Barberi G, Galván González FJ, Miranda Fernández S, Viera Peláez D, Medina Rivero F, Marrero Saavedra D. Vasoproliferative retinopathy secondary to Waldenström's disease. Arch Soc Esp Oftalmol. 2019;94(2):85–9. English, Spanish. https://doi.org/10.1016/j.oftal.2018.09.006.
40. Gertz MA. Acute hyperviscosity: syndromes and management. Blood. 2018;132:1379–85. https://doi.org/10.1182/blood-2018-06-846816.
41. Hill QA, Stamps R, Massey E, Grainger JD, Provan D, Hill A. The diagnosis and management of primary autoimmune haemolytic anaemia. Br J Haematol. 2017;176(3):395–411. https://doi.org/10.1111/bjh.14478.
42. Michalak SS, Olewicz-Gawlik A, Rupa-Matysek J, Wolny-Rokicka E, Nowakowska E, Gil L. Autoimmune hemolytic anemia: current knowledge and perspectives. Immun Ageing. 2020;17(1):38. https://doi.org/10.1186/s12979-020-00208-7.
43. Cacoub P, Vieira M, Saadoun D. Cryoglobulinemia - one name for two diseases. N Engl J Med. 2024;391:1426–39. http://www.ncbi.nlm.nih.gov/pubmed/39413378
44. Dammacco F, Lauletta G, Vacca A. The wide spectrum of cryoglobulinemic vasculitis and an overview of therapeutic advancements. Clin Exp Med. 2023;23(2):255–72. https://doi.org/10.1007/s10238-022-00808-1.
45. Quartuccio L, Bortoluzzi A, Scirè CA, Marangoni A, Del Frate G, Treppo E, et al. Management of mixed cryoglobulinemia with rituximab: evidence and consensus-based recommendations from the Italian Study Group of Cryoglobulinemia (GISC). Clin Rheumatol. 2023;42(2):359–70. https://doi.org/10.1007/s10067-022-06391-w.
46. Miao J, Krisanapan P, Tangpanithandee S, Thongprayoon C, Cheungpasitporn W. Efficacy of therapeutic apheresis for cryoglobulinemic vasculitis patients with renal involvement: a systematic review. Blood Purif. 2024;53:1–9. https://doi.org/10.1159/000534102.
47. Zhu P, Wu Y, et al. ABO-incompatible allogeneic hematopoietic stem cell transplantation. Blood Genom. 2023;7(1):1–12. https://doi.org/10.46701/BG.2023012022036.
48. Vaezi M, Dameshghi DO, Souri M, Setarehdan SA, Alimoghaddam K, Ghavamzadeh A. ABO incompatibility and hematopoietic stem cell

transplantation outcomes. Int J Hematol Stem Cell Res. 2017;11(2):139–47.

49. Gladstone DE, Bettinotti MP. HLA donor-specific antibodies in allogeneic hematopoietic stem cell transplantation: challenges and opportunities. Hematology. 2017;2017(1):645–50. https://doi.org/10.1182/asheducation-2017.1.645.
50. Garnett C, Apperley JF, Pavlu J. Treatment and management of graft-versus-host disease: improving response and survival. Ther Adv Hematol. 2013;4(6):366–78. https://doi.org/10.1177/2040620713489842.
51. Filipovich AH, Weisdorf D, Pavletic S, Socie G, Wingard JR, Lee SJ, et al. National Institutes of Health consensus development project on criteria for clinical trials in chronic graft-versus-host disease: I. Diagnosis and staging working group report. Biol Blood Marrow Transplant. 2005;11(12):945–56. https://doi.org/10.1016/j.bbmt.2005.09.004.
52. Asensi Cantó P, Sanz Caballer J, Solves Alcaína P, de la Rubia CJ, Gómez SI. Extracorporeal photopheresis in graft-versus-host disease. Transplant Cell Ther. 2023;29(9):556–66. https://doi.org/10.1016/j.jtct.2023.07.001.
53. Elendu C, Amaechi DC, Alakwe-Ojimba CE, Elendu TC, Elendu RC, Ayabazu CP, et al. Understanding sickle cell disease: causes, symptoms, and treatment options. Medicine. 2023;102(38):e35237. https://doi.org/10.1097/MD.0000000000035237.
54. Brandow AM, Liem RI. Advances in the diagnosis and treatment of sickle cell disease. J Hematol Oncol. 2022;15(1):20. https://doi.org/10.1186/s13045-022-01237-z.
55. Mithoowani S, Laureano M, Crowther MA, Hillis CM. Investigation and management of erythrocytosis. CMAJ. 2020;192(32):E913–8. https://doi.org/10.1503/cmaj.191587.
56. Bleeker JS, Hogan WJ. Thrombocytosis: diagnostic evaluation, thrombotic risk stratification, and risk-based management strategies. Thromb. 2011;2:011:536062. https://doi.org/10.1155/2011/536062.
57. Röllig C, Ehninger G. How I treat hyperleukocytosis in acute myeloid leukemia. Blood. 2015;125(21):3246–52. https://doi.org/10.1182/blood-2014-10-551507.
58. Aqui N, O'Doherty U. Leukocytapheresis for the treatment of hyperleukocytosis secondary to acute leukemia. Hematol (United States). 2014;2014(1):457–60. https://doi.org/10.1182/asheducation-2014.1.457.

Indications for PEX: Rheumatology

5

Abstract

Autoantibodies and immune complexes play a pivotal role in the pathogenesis of a wide range of rheumatic diseases. Therapeutic apheresis removes these pathogenic molecules from plasma. Several apheresis modalities are used in rheumatology. However, their role as treatment option has evolved with the introduction of novel immunosuppressive and anti-inflammatory agents (e.g., Rituximab, Infliximab). This chapter will demonstrate different apheresis protocols in major rheumatic diseases (e.g., systemic lupus erythematosus, ANCA-associated vasculitis, catastrophic antiphospholipid syndrome) and will discuss their effectiveness in association with current pharmacological therapies.

Keywords

ANCA-associated vasculitis · Systemic lupus erythematosus (SLE) · Catastrophic antiphospholipid syndrome (CAPS)

ANCA-Associated Vasculitis

Definition Antineutrophil cytoplasmic antibody (ANCA)-associated vasculitis (AAV) is a disease, associated with necrotizing inflammatory process predominantly of small vessels

J. J. Filipov, *Therapeutic Plasma Exchange*, In Clinical Practice, https://doi.org/10.1007/978-3-032-17275-4_5

(arterioles, capillaries and venules), without deposition of immune complexes. It encompasses three subtypes—granulomatosis with polyangiitis (GMP), microscopic polyangiitis (MPA), and eosinophilic granulomatosis with polyangiitis (EGP) [1]. GMP and MPA account for approximately 80–90% of all AAV [2]. AAV affects multiple organs and systems, and clinical presentation may overlap between different types of AAV. However, EGP rarely involves lungs and kidneys [3]. In addition, limited kidney involvement is also present, characterized with necrotizing crescentic glomerulonephritis.

Pathogenesis and pathophysiology AAV pathogenesis is multifactorial. Genetic predisposition (Caucasians, HLA-DRB1*15, HLA-DRB1*1101, and DRB1*1202 alleles), as well as environmental factors (silica dust, farming, Staphylococcus aureus carriage) have been established [2, 4]. Neutrophils (Neu) play a pivotal role in AAV, as ANCA-activated Neu cause degranulation, cytokine release, and endothelial damage. Additionally, proinflammatory cytokines, complement activation, and T cell dysregulation are involved in AAV pathogenesis [4].

Clinical presentation Granulomatous inflammation is typical for GMP and is not present in MPA. Multiple systems are involved and symptoms may overlap between different AAV subtypes [2]:

- General symptoms—fever, weight loss, myalgia, arthralgia
- CNS—cranial nerve palsy, CNS meningitis, ischemia/hemorrhagic events
- Peripheral nervous system—mononeuritis multiplex, polyneuropathy
- Upper airways—mucosal inflammation; presence of nasal septum perforation—typical for GMP
- Lungs—pulmonary infiltrates, diffuse alveolar hemorrhage, nodules with cavities (GMP), pleural effusions
- Ocular symptoms—conjunctivitis, scleritis, etc.
- Heart—coronary disease, arrhythmia

- Gastrointestinal tract—bleeding, diarrhea, pancreatitis, hepatitis
- Kidneys—rapidly progressive glomerulonephritis
- Skin—palpable purpura, nodules, livedo reticularis

Laboratory findings usually confirm organ involvement (e.g., kidneys, liver, heart); imaging demonstrates lung (chest X-ray/chest CT scan) or CNS involvement. Immunology for ANCA demonstrates AAV; anti-MPO autoantibodies are more frequently detected in MPA, whereas anti-PR3 antibodies are usually associated with GMP. The presence of one type of ANCA usually excludes the presence of the other. In addition, anti-GBM antibodies can be detected, which is linked to poorer outcomes. Rarely, testing for both ANCA subtypes can be negative, necessitating additional diagnostic evaluation; seronegative vasculitis has unclear pathogenesis, but other autoantibodies have been suggested; its clinical presentation may differ from AAV; in seronegative forms, renal-limited involvement is more frequently detected and extrarenal manifestations are less frequently established [5].

Generally, organ biopsy (kidney, lung, muscle) is regarded as the golden standard for AAV diagnosis (Photo 5.1). However, in the presence of positive ANCA testing and corresponding clinical presentation, organ biopsy may not be mandatory [6].

Treatment of AAV Two major aspects of AAV treatment are present: remission induction and maintenance therapy.

Induction therapy consists of high-dose steroids, combined with RTX and/or Cyclophosphamide. Different dosing regimens have been suggested for both steroids and immunosuppressive therapy. RTX is preferred in AAV relapse. Once remission has been achieved for 3–6 months, maintenance treatment is initiated [2]. In milder AAV, other medications can be used in combination with steroids—azathioprine, mycophenolate mofetil, Avacopan, and methotrexate.

Maintenance treatment usually lasts for 24–48 months and consists of steroid dose reduction and RTX; Azathioprine and methotrexate can be used alternatively [7].

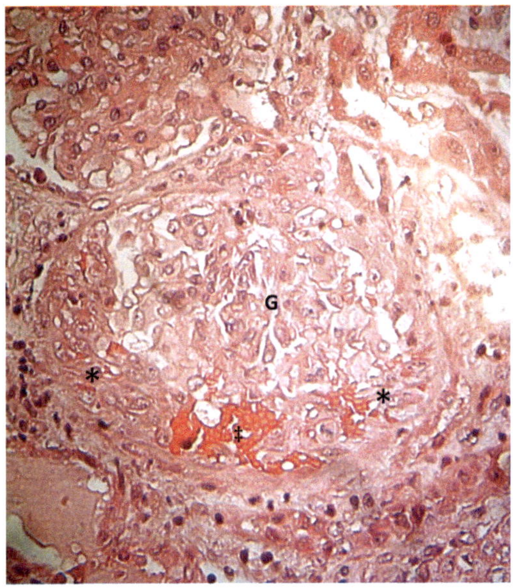

Photo 5.1 Kidney involvement in ANCA vasculitis, anti-MPO /+/ positive. Hematoxylin eosin staining, magnification x250. Cellular crescent and RBC extravasation of red blood cells are detected. *—cellular crescent; ‡—extravasation of red blood cells; G—glomerular tuft. (Photo courtesy Assoc.-Prof. Todorov, Department of General and Clinical Pathology, Medical University—Sofia, Bulgaria)

PEX in the treatment of AAV PEX is currently not recommended as routine therapy in AAV. Though earlier studies demonstrated benefit from PEX, the PEXIVAS study failed to establish improved outcomes in AAV patients treated with PEX (incidence of death or end-stage kidney disease, ESKD), both in advanced kidney injury or diffuse alveolar hemorrhage (DAH) [8]. A recent meta-analysis also failed to establish significant benefit from PEX in AAV-associated DAH. The same study demonstrated reduced end-stage renal disease incidence at 12 month after treatment in the PEX group; however, PEX-treated patient had higher incidence of infection [9].

KDIGO suggests that PEX should be considered in AAV and serum creatinine >300 µmol/l (>3.4 mg/dl), rapidly decreasing kidney function, dialysis-dependent patients, or hypoxemic DAH [1]. European League Against Rheumatism (EULAR) does not recommend the routine use of PEX in DAH, but it may be considered in active glomerulonephritis and serum creatinine >300 µmol/l (>3.4 mg/dl) [7]. Finally, the routine use of PEX is not recommended by the American College of Rheumatology (ACR) too; it may be used in AAV patients with increased risk for ESKD, who accept potential risk of infection [10]. The use of PEX in AAV falls into ASFA category 3, indicating unclear benefit of the treatment [3].

The following PEX schedule is suggested:

- Treatment volume per PEX: 1–1.5 EPV.
- Interval between PEX procedures: 24 h (DAH), 48 h (without DAH).
- Substitution fluid: human albumin; FFP in DAH.
- End of treatment: Generally, until symptoms resolve. In patients with severe kidney involvement without DAH—usually 7 PEX over 14 days. In AAV-associated DAH—daily PEX until pulmonary bleeding stops.

In cases of double positivity (ANCA /+/ positive, anti-GBM /+/ positive), treatment should be performed as in anti-GBM disease—see section "Anti-glomerular Basement Membrane (Anti-GBM) Disease" , Chap. 3 of this book.

Systemic Lupus Erythematosus (SLE)

Definition SLE is an autoimmune disease affecting multiple organs and systems. It has a chronic course with flare-ups, and is associated with autoantibodies to nuclear and cytoplasmic antigens, though autoantibodies specific for other conditions can be detected (e.g., systemic sclerosis, Sjogren syndrome), indicating its association to other autoimmune diseases.

Pathogenesis and pathophysiology The pathogenesis of SLE is multifactorial. It is generally recognized that environmental factors trigger autoimmune response in genetically predisposed individuals [11]. A wide range of environmental factors have been detected—ultraviolet light, infectious agents (e.g., Epstein-Barr infection, EBV), toxins (silica dust, heavy metals, smoking), and drugs (e.g., hydralazine, procainamide); it is believed that they can induce systemic autoimmunity by causing cell damage and exposure to autoantigens [12]. Additionally, hormonal factors—estrogen production/estrogen-based medications—can cause SLE flares. A large number of genetic polymorphisms were identified, linked to polygenic and monogenic SLE forms; these genetic polymorphisms encode lymphocyte and type 1 interferon signaling as well as clearance of immune complexes [11].

Several immunological abnormalities in SLE were detected: dysregulated interferon 1 production, overproduction of pro-inflammatory cytokines, impaired T cell balance, impaired debris clearance. The latter is of particular importance—dying cells release autoantigens, which are normally fully removed by immune complexes (consisting of autoantigens and antibodies against them) and no inflammation occurs; however, in SLE due to their inadequate removal, immune complexes are being deposited in different organs, amplifying immune response and causing further cellular damage [13].

Clinical presentation As the presentation of SLE may involve various systems and organs, different diagnostic criteria have been used over the years; recently, the EULAR/ACR Classification Criteria for Systemic Lupus Erythematosus have been published [14]:

A. Entry criterion—positive testing for antinuclear antibodies (ANA)
B. Clinical criteria
   - Constitutional: fever
   - Hematologic: leucopenia, thrombocytopenia, autoimmune hemolysis

- CNS involvement: psychosis, delirium, seizures
- Mucosal/skin involvement: non-scarring alopecia, acute/subacute cutaneous lupus, discoid lupus
- Serosal: pleural/pericardial effusions, acute pericarditis
- Musculoskeletal: joint involvement
- Kidney involvement: proteinuria >0.5 grams/24 h, lupus nephritis types 2–5 on kidney biopsy

C. Immunological criteria
- Presence of antiphospholipid antibodies: anti-cardiolipin antibodies or anti-β2GP1 antibodies or lupus anticoagulant
- Complement testing: low C3 and/or low C4
- Presence of SLE specific antibodies: anti-double-stranded DNA (ant-ds DNA) antibody or anti-Smith (anti-Sm) antibody

Criteria for groups B and C have different weight, expressed in number of points for each criterion. SLE classification requires positive entry criterion—positive test for ANA. Once entry criterion is present, SLE diagnosis requires at least one clinical criterion (group B) and total score ≥10 points.

Additionally, different algorithms for assessing disease activity were introduced into clinical practice (e.g., SLEDAI and BILAG scoring systems) [13].

Treatment of SLE Treatment of SLE varies according to disease activity and organ involvement. Generally, hydroxychloroquine is recommended in all patients, if no contraindications exist. Steroids can be used as maintenance doses; however, in moderate or severe disease, pulse steroids should be used. Immunomodulating/immunosuppressive agents (e.g., methotrexate, azathioprine, or mycophenolate) and/or biological agents (e.g., belimumab, anifrolumab) can be added to the treatment if no effect from steroids and hydroxychloroquine is present. In organ-/life-threatening cases, high-dose intravenous cyclophosphamyde/RTX should be considered. Calcineurin inhibitors can be added to the therapy of lupus nephritis. In antiphospholipid syndrome, vitamin K antagonists and low-dose acetyl salicylic acid are recommended [15].

PEX in the management of SLE Therapeutic apheresis (PEX, IA) is not recommended as first-line treatment for induction or maintenance [3]. Its use is supported in cases of life−/organ-threatening SLE, not responding to recommended immunosuppressive treatment [e.g., catastrophic antiphospholipid syndrome (CAPS); thrombotic microangiopathy, especially SLE-associated thrombotic thrombocytopenic purpura; cryoglobulinemia; DAH; CNS involvement; hyperviscosity; leucopenia; thrombocytopenia] [15–17].

Generally, a more intensive PEX regimen is used for lupus nephritis (LN) and DAH [3].

- Treatment volume per procedure: 1–1.5 EPV.
- Substitution fluid: human albumin/FFP; FFP in TMA (especially TTP) and CAPS.
- Interval between procedures: 24 or 48 h (LN, DAH); three procedures weekly for other complications. For TMA/CAPS daily PEX is required.
- End of treatment: achieved clinical improvement.

Catastrophic Antiphospholipid Syndrome (CAPS)

Definition Antiphospholipid syndrome (APS) is a thrombotic-inflammatory disease, mediated by antiphospholipid antibodies (lupus anticoagulant, anti-cardiolipin antibodies. or antiβ2 glycoprotein I antibodies), manifesting with vascular thromboses and recurrent miscarriages. A more severe form of APS, causing organ failure, is the catastrophic APS (CAPS), defined as the presence of organ/tissue/system failure (at least 3 involved); occurring simultaneously or within 7 days, with positive test for antiphospholipid antibodies and confirmed small vessel occlusion on histology [18]. APS can be primary, but secondary forms, associated with autoimmune diseases (especially SLE) are also present.

Pathogenesis and pathophysiology Several pathogenic factors are involved in APS—autoantibodies against phospholipids and beta 2 glycoprotein I, T cell dysregulation, and genetic predisposition. Thrombus formation can be associated with 2-hit model—first hit is the presence of antiphospholipid antibodies and the second hit is vascular injury or inflammation. Additionally, complement dysregulation may also play a role in APS [19].

Clinical presentation APS presents with venous and arterial thromboses, involving all locations, but most commonly affecting deep veins of lower extremities and cerebral arteries. Obstetric manifestations include recurrent early miscarriage or pre-eclampsia. CAPS is a life-threatening form of APS, presenting with organ/tissue/system failure (at least 3 involved), occurring simultaneously or within 7 days, with positive test for antiphospholipid antibodies and confirmed small vessel occlusion on histology. Additionally, APS may present with non-criteria manifestations, such as cardiac valve damage, antiphospholipid antibody-associated nephropathy, diffuse alveolar hemorrhage (DAH), thrombocytopenia, and livedo reticularis. Laboratory testing should include antiphospholipid antibodies, as well as immunology for SLE; triple positivity for all three types of APS antibody tests (anti-β2GPI antibodies, anti-cardiolipin antibodies, lupus anticoagulant test) is associated with higher risk for thrombotic events [19].

Treatment of APS and CAPS. Role of PEX Generally, in APS anticoagulation with vitamin K antagonists is recommended; in recurrent arterial thrombosis, low molecular heparins can be used. In obstetric APS, prophylaxis with low-dose Aspirin or/and heparin is recommended [20]. CAPS can be triggered by infections, surgical procedures, and anticoagulant prophylaxis discontinuation in previously known APS. First-line treatment consists of triple combination: steroids, heparin, PEX or intravenous immunoglobulin (IVIG), or PEX + IVIG. In refractory CAPS RTX, eculisumab and cyclophosphamide may be added to the treatment as second-line agents [18, 20]. ASFA guidelines also categorize PEX as first-line treatment, in combination with steroids and heparin (ASFA category 1). The following treatment schedule is recommended [3]:

- Treatment volume per PEX: 1.0–1.5 EPV
- Interval between procedures: 24–48 h
- Substitution fluid: FFP or FFP + albumin
- End of treatment: resolution of symptoms; consider antiphospholipid antibody titers monitoring

Systemic Sclerosis

Definition Systemic sclerosis (SSC) is a chronic autoimmune connective tissue disease characterized by vasculopathy and subsequent progressive organ fibrosis and organ failure. It has multifactorial pathogenesis and a wide range of clinical symptoms and is associated with increased mortality [21].

Pathogenesis and pathophysiology Similar to other autoimmune diseases, in the pathogenesis of SSC, a wide range of factors play a significant role. Environmental factors [silica professional exposure, viral infections (CMV, EBV, Human herpes virus 6)] can trigger chronic autoimmune and inflammatory process in genetically predisposed (HLA, STAT4, IRF5, and CD247 genetic variants) individuals. Immune dysregulation is a key factor in SSC, as abnormalities in macrophages, neutrophils, dendrite cells were described, as well as T- and B cell dysregulation; SSC-specific autoantibodies also were detected, e.g., anti-centromere (ACA), anti-topoisomerase I (anti-SCL 70), and anti-RNA polymerase antibodies. Vasculopathy, probably initiated by immune dysregulation, consisting of endothelial cell damage, dysfunction, and defective remodeling, is a pivotal pathogenic mechanism. Vasculopathy causes chronic inflammation, chronic tissue injury, which progresses to fibrosis and organ failure [21, 22].

Clinical Presentation and Laboratory Findings

Clinically SSC has various clinical manifestations and may be part of overlap syndromes [23]:

- Raynaud phenomenon
- Skin involvement: according to the areas affected, skin damage is classified as limited (distal to the elbows and knees) and dif-

fuse (proximal to the elbows, knees, and/or the trunk). Initially, inflammation of the involved regions occurs, followed by skin thickening and fibrosis. Progression of skin fibrosis causes contractures. Additionally, depigmentation, skin ulcers, telangiectasias, and subcutaneous calcinosis may be detected.

- Musculoskeletal involvement: inflammatory arthritis, osteolysis, muscle fibrosis, and atrophy.
- Gastrointestinal involvement: perioral skin fibrosis, periodontitis, gingivitis, esophageal dysmotility, gastroparesis, and intestinal dysmotility.
- Pulmonary involvement: most typically interstitial lung disease and pulmonary arterial hypertension (PAH).
- Cardiac involvement: pericardial effusions, dilated cardiomiopathy, and arrhythmias.
- Renal involvement: Scleroderma renal crisis (SRC) due to SSC vasculopathy of renal vessels, presenting with hypertension and impaired kidney function. Additionally, hematuria, proteinuria, and thrombotic microangiopathy may be detected.

Specific laboratory findings include the detection of the following autoantibodies: Anti-centromere Ab, Anti-topoisomerase I (Scl-70) Ab, Anti-RNA polymerase III Ab, though other autoantibodies can also be detected.

Treatment of SSC Dihydropiridine calcium blockers and phosphodiesterase-5 inhibitors (PDE5i) are used for the treatment of Raynaud phenomenon. PDE5i and iloprost are recommended in digital ulcers. Endothelin receptor antagonists and PDE5i are recommended in PAH. ACE inhibitors are recommended as first-line treatment of SRC. Immunosuppression (cyclophosphamide, RTX, metotrexate, mycophenolates) are recommended in diffuse skin SSC and interstitial lung disease [24].

Role of therapeutic apheresis in SSC Two types of therapeutic apheresis were used in SSC - ECP and PEX; their benefit still is unclear (ASFA category 3) and more studies are rquired.

ECP, performed 1 cycle (2 procedures in 2 consecutive days) every 4–6 weeks, over 6–12 months, demonstrated improvement in skin involvement; however, data demonstrate relatively short-lasting effect [25].

PEX demonstrated improved outcomes in SRC with TMA, as well as Raynaud syndrome and digital ulceration. Maintenance PEX treatment may be needed.

ECP treatment in SSC [3]:

- Treatment schedule: 1 treatment cycle every 4–6 weeks, for 6–12 months
- End of treatment: re-evaluate at sixth month, if no improvement—consider cessation of treatment

PEX in SSC [3]:

- Treatment volume per PEX: 1.0–1.5 EPV
- Interval between procedures: 48–72 h; 2–3 PEX per week over 4 weeks
- Substitution fluid: albumin
- End of treatment: improvement in symptoms, serum creatinine stabilization.

Other Rheumatic Diseases

Idiopathic Polyarteritis Nodosa (PANi)

PANi is a systemic necrotizing inflammation of medium size arteries, presenting with wide range of affected organs (peripheral neuropathy, renovascular hypertension, abdominal pain, skin nodules). The disease is diagnosed by organ biopsy or angiography. Current treatment includes immunosuppression (steroids + cyclophosphamide, methotrexate, mycophenolic acid derivatives). PEX is not recommended in iPAN, it was categorized as ASFA category 4 in previous editions of the ASFA guidelines and is not included in the latest ones as no new evidence appeared [26, 27].

Hepatitis B Virus (HBV)-Associated PAN

HBV-associated PAN is a necrotizing inflammation of medium size arteries, secondary to HBV infection. The pathogenesis of HVB-associated PAN is related to deposition of immune complexes, which trigger endothelial inflammation. Treatment of HBV-associated PAN consists of high-dose steroids, anti-viral medications, and PEX as adjunctive therapy (ASFA category 2). The following PEX schedule in HBV-PAN is suggested [3, 28]:

- Treatment volume per PEX: 1.0–1.5 EPV
- Substitution: albumin
- PEX scheme: 3 procedures weekly (over 3 weeks), followed by 2 PEX weekly for 2 weeks, followed by 1 PEX per week
- End of treatment: resolution of symptoms for 2 months; seroconversion from HBV E antigen to HBV E–antibody

Rheumatoid Arthritis

Rheumatoid arthritis is a systemic autoimmune disease, affecting predominantly small joints; however, extra-articular involvement (lungs, ocular disturbances) is also possible. Treatment relies on disease-modifying antirheumatic drugs (biological, synthetic), as well as steroids. PEX is not indicated in rheumatoid arthritis (ASFA category 4) [29].

Dermatomyositis and Polymyositis

Dermatomyositis and polymyositis represent different types of inflammatory myopathy, presenting with muscle weakness, but it can affect also lungs and gastrointestinal tract. The etiology of the disease is unclear, but genetic predisposition, as well as malignancies and other environmental factors may play a role in the pathogenesis. Currently, treatment includes steroids and immunosuppressive treatment (azathioprine, methotrexate, and tacrolimus). Therapeutic apheresis (ECP, PEX) is not recommended in the treatment of dermatomyositis and polymyositis (ASFA category 4) [30, 31].

References

1. Floege J, Jayne DRW, Sanders JSF, Tesar V, Rovin BH. KDIGO 2024 clinical practice guideline for the management of antineutrophil cytoplasmic antibody (ANCA)–associated vasculitis. Kidney Int. 2024;105(3S):S71–S116. https://doi.org/10.1016/j.kint.2023.10.008.
2. Chevet B, Cornec D, Casal Moura M, Cornec-Le Gall E, Fervenza FC, Warrington KJ, et al. Diagnosing and treating ANCA-associated vasculitis: an updated review for clinical practice. Rheumatology. 2023;62(5):1787–803. https://doi.org/10.1093/rheumatology/keac623.
3. Connelly-Smith L, Alquist CR, Aqui NA, Hofmann JC, Klingel R, Onwuemene OA, et al. Guidelines on the use of therapeutic apheresis in clinical practice – evidence-based approach from the writing Committee of the American Society for Apheresis: the ninth special issue. J Clin Apher. 2023;38(2):77–278. https://doi.org/10.1002/jca.22043.
4. Xiao H, Hu P, Falk RJ, Jennette JC. Overview of the pathogenesis of ANCA-associated vasculitis. Kidney Dis. 2015;1(4):205–15. https://doi.org/10.1159/000442323.
5. Juanet C, Hassi I, Koirala A. ANCA-negative Pauci-immune glomerulonephritis: a review. Glomerular Dis. 2024;4(1):189–99. https://doi.org/10.1159/000541792.
6. Suppiah R, Robson JC, Grayson PC, Ponte C, Craven A, Khalid S, et al. 2022 American college of rheumatology/European alliance of associations for rheumatology classification criteria for microscopic polyangiitis. Ann Rheum Dis. 2022;81(3):321–6. https://doi.org/10.1136/annrheumdis-2021-221796.
7. Hellmich B, Sanchez-Alamo B, Schirmer JH, Berti A, Blockmans D, Cid MC, et al. EULAR recommendations for the management of ANCA-associated vasculitis: 2022 update. Ann Rheum Dis. 2023;83(1):30–47. https://doi.org/10.1136/ard-2022-223764.
8. Walsh M, Merkel PA, Peh C-A, Szpirt WM, Puéchal X, Fujimoto S, et al. Plasma exchange and glucocorticoids in severe ANCA-associated vasculitis. N Engl J Med. 2020;382(7):622–31. https://doi.org/10.1056/NEJMoa1803537.
9. Walsh M, Collister D, Zeng L, Merkel PA, Pusey CD, Guyatt G, et al. The effects of plasma exchange in patients with ANCA-associated vasculitis:

an updated systematic review and meta-analysis. BMJ. 2022;376:e064604. https://doi.org/10.1136/bmj-2021-064604.

10. Chung SA, Langford CA, Maz M, Abril A, Gorelik M, Guyatt G, et al. 2021 American College of Rheumatology/Vasculitis Foundation guideline for the management of antineutrophil cytoplasmic antibody–associated vasculitis. Arthritis Rheumatol. 2021;73:1366–83. https://doi.org/10.1002/art.41773.
11. Ameer MA, Chaudhry H, Mushtaq J, Khan OS, Babar M, Hashim T, et al. An overview of systemic lupus erythematosus (SLE) pathogenesis, classification, and management. Cureus. 2022;14(10):e30330. https://doi.org/10.7759/cureus.30330.
12. Woo JMP, Parks CG, Jacobsen S, Costenbader KH, Bernatsky S. The role of environmental exposures and gene–environment interactions in the etiology of systemic lupus erythematous. J Intern Med. 2022;291:755–78. https://doi.org/10.1111/joim.13448.
13. Dai X, Fan Y, Zhao X. Systemic lupus erythematosus: updated insights on the pathogenesis, diagnosis, prevention and therapeutics. Signal Transduct Target Ther [Internet]. 2025;10:102. https://doi.org/10.1038/s41392-025-02168-0.
14. Aringer M, Costenbader K, Daikh D, Brinks R, Mosca M, Ramsey-Goldman R, et al. 2019 European league against rheumatism/American College of Rheumatology classification criteria for systemic lupus erythematosus. Ann Rheum Dis. 2019;71(9):1400–12. https://doi.org/10.1002/art.40930.
15. Fanouriakis A, Kostopoulou M, Andersen J, Aringer M, Arnaud L, Bae SC, et al. EULAR recommendations for the management of systemic lupus erythematosus: 2023 update. Ann Rheum Dis. 2023;83(1):15–29. https://doi.org/10.1136/ard-2023-224762.
16. Kidney Disease: Improving Global Outcomes (KDIGO) Lupus Nephritis Work Group. KDIGO 2024 clinical practice guideline for the management of Lupus Nephritis. Kidney Int. 2024;105(1S):S1–S69. https://doi.org/10.1016/j.kint.2023.09.002.
17. Gordon C, Amissah-Arthur MB, Gayed M, Brown S, Bruce IN, D'Cruz D, et al. The British Society for Rheumatology guideline for the management of systemic lupus erythematosus in adults. Rheumatology. 2018;57(1):e1–e45. https://doi.org/10.1093/rheumatology/kex286.
18. Ambati A, Knight JS, Zuo Y. Antiphospholipid syndrome management: a 2023 update and practical algorithm-based approach. Curr Opin Rheumatol. 2023;35(3):149–60. https://doi.org/10.1097/BOR.0000000000000932.
19. Knight JS, Branch DW, Ortel TL. Antiphospholipid syndrome: advances in diagnosis, pathogenesis, and management. BMJ. 2023;380:e069717. https://doi.org/10.1136/bmj-2021-069717.
20. Tektonidou MG, Andreoli L, Limper M, Amoura Z, Cervera R, Costedoat-Chalumeau N, et al. EULAR recommendations for the management of

antiphospholipid syndrome in adults. Ann Rheum Dis. 2019;78(10):1296–304. https://doi.org/10.1136/annrheumdis-2019-215213.

21. Son HH, Moon SJ. Pathogenesis of systemic sclerosis: an integrative review of recent advances. J Rheum Dis. 2025;32:89–104. https://doi.org/10.4078/jrd.2024.0129.
22. Benfaremo D, Svegliati S, Paolini C, Agarbati S, Moroncini G. Systemic sclerosis: from pathophysiology to novel therapeutic approaches. Biomedicine. 2022;10(1):163. https://doi.org/10.3390/biomedicines10010163.
23. Van Den Hoogen F, Khanna D, Fransen J, Johnson SR, Baron M, Tyndall A, et al. 2013 classification criteria for systemic sclerosis: an American college of rheumatology/European league against rheumatism collaborative initiative. Arthritis Rheum. 2013;65(11):2737–47. https://doi.org/10.1002/art.38098.
24. Del Galdo F, Lescoat A, Conaghan PG, Bertoldo E, Čolić J, Santiago T, et al. EULAR recommendations for the treatment of systemic sclerosis: 2023 update. Ann Rheum Dis. 2025;84(1):29–40. https://doi.org/10.1136/ard-2024-226430.
25. Papp G, Horvath IF, Gyimesi E, Barath S, Vegh J, Szodoray P, et al. The assessment of immune-regulatory effects of extracorporeal photopheresis in systemic sclerosis: a long-term follow-up study. Immunol Res. 2016;64(2):404–11. https://doi.org/10.1007/s12026-015-8678-5.
26. Padmanabhan A, Connelly-Smith L, Aqui N, Balogun RA, Klingel R, Meyer E, et al. Guidelines on the use of therapeutic apheresis in clinical practice - evidence-based approach from the writing Committee of the American Society for Apheresis: the eighth special issue. J Clin Apher. 2019;34:171–354. https://doi.org/10.1002/jca.21705.
27. Chung SA, Gorelik M, Langford CA, Maz M, Abril A, Guyatt G, et al. 2021 American College of Rheumatology/Vasculitis Foundation guideline for the management of polyarteritis nodosa. Arthritis Care Res. 2021;73(8):1061–70. https://doi.org/10.1002/acr.24633.
28. Guillevin L, Mahr A, Callard P, Godmer P, Pagnoux C, Leray E, et al. Hepatitis B virus-associated polyarteritis nodosa: clinical characteristics, outcome, and impact of treatment in 115 patients. Medicine (Baltimore). 2005;84(5):313–22. https://doi.org/10.1097/01.md.0000180792.80212.5e.
29. Szczepiorkowski ZM, Winters JL, Bandarenko N, Kim HC, Linenberger ML, Marques MB, et al. Guidelines on the use of therapeutic apheresis in clinical practice - evidence-based approach from the apheresis applications committee of the American Society for Apheresis. J Clin Apher. 2010;25(3):83–177. https://doi.org/10.1002/jca.20240.

30. Kohsaka H, Mimori T, Kanda T, Shimizu J, Sunada Y, Fujimoto M, et al. Treatment consensus for management of polymyositis and dermatomyositis among rheumatologists, neurologists and dermatologists. Mod Rheumatol. 2019;29(1):1–19. https://doi.org/10.1080/14397595.2018.1521185.
31. Schwartz J, Padmanabhan A, Aqui N, Balogun RA, Connelly-Smith L, Delaney M, et al. Guidelines on the use of therapeutic apheresis in clinical practice—evidence-based approach from the writing Committee of the American Society for Apheresis: the seventh special issue. J Clin Apher. 2016;31(3):149–62. https://doi.org/10.1002/jca.21470.

Indications for PEX: Neurology

6

Abstract

Autoimmunity plays a pivotal role in a wide range of neurological disorders, affecting the peripheral and central nervous system. Removal of autoantibodies by different therapeutic apheresis modalities (PEX, DFPP, IA) remains the major treatment option in certain neurological diseases (e.g., acute inflammatory demyelinating polyradiculoneuropathy, acute myasthenia gravis, resistant acute disseminated encephalopathy). Despite the introduction of novel immunosuppressive agents (IVIG, RTX), which have also improved the outcomes in autoimmune neurological conditions, PEX is of particular importance in acute severe episodes of the diseases, where rapid clinical improvement is needed. The aim of this chapter is to demonstrate the effectiveness of therapeutic apheresis in neurological pathology in the light of modern treatment options.

Keywords

Multiple sclerosis · N-Methyl-D-Aspartate Receptor Antibody (NMDARA) Encephalitis · Guillain-Barré syndrome · Myasthenia gravis

J. J. Filipov, *Therapeutic Plasma Exchange*, In Clinical Practice,
https://doi.org/10.1007/978-3-032-17275-4_6

Diseases of the Central Nervous System

Multiple Sclerosis

Definition Multiple sclerosis (MS) is a chronic inflammatory disease, affecting the central nervous system. MS usually affects young adults and presents with visual loss, muscle weakness, sensory deficits, and typical MRI lesions [1].

Pathogenesis and pathophysiology Several environmental factors were identified with increased risk for MS: infections (EBV, human herpes virus type 6), smoking, ultraviolet radiation, and vitamin deficits (D, B12). Environmental factors may trigger inflammation in genetically predisposed individuals (e.g., HLA genetic variants), which leads to immune dysregulation and inflammation of white and grey matter. The inflammatory process also impairs myelin reparation in MS [2].

Clinical presentation MS symptoms are heterogeneous and may include visual disturbances (visual loss, double vision), vestibular (ataxia) and bulbar (dysarthria and dysphagia) symptoms, muscle weakness, sensory dysfunction, genitourinary (incontinence and retention), and gastrointestinal (constipation, diarrhea). Characteristic findings on brain MRI are used to diagnose MS. Different clinical patterns are present in MS [3]:

- Relapsing-remitting MS: Presents with acute episodes of the above-mentioned neurological symptoms, occurring within days/weeks and lasting for 24–48 h. The patient is relatively stable between episodes, but residual symptoms remain, leading to disability.
- Primary–progressive MS: The disease has initially progressive course, without episodes of exacerbations.
- Secondary progressive MS: Secondary to relapsing-remitting form, MS evolves to slowly progressive disease.

- Relapsing-progressive MS: Gradual progression of the disease, accompanied by episodes of relapse.
- Clinically isolated syndrome: Single isolated episode of neurological symptoms.

Treatment of MS Treatment consists of disease-modifying treatment and treatment of acute attack/relapse. Disease modifying treatment aims at slowing down MS progression and prevention of relapses. Several preparations are used (e.g., β-interferons, monoclonal antibodies, glatiramer acetate, and fingolimod). Acute relapses are treated with pulse steroids; however, if there is no improvement after 2 weeks of steroid initiation, PEX should be considered. Alternatively, second steroid pulse, intravenous immunoglobulins (IVIG), RTX, and cyclophosphamide can be used [4].

PEX in the treatment of MS Two types of therapeutic apheresis modalities can be used in MS –PEX and IA. Both PEX and IA are second-line treatment in acute relapses in relapsing-remitting MS; PEX/IA are used in refractory MS episodes, without clinical improvement after 14 days from steroid pulse initiation. The two types of therapeutic apheresis have similar effectiveness and safety profile [5]. PEX and IA can be used in acute MS relapse in pregnant women. In progressive MS forms, PEX/IA are generally regarded ineffective; they may be considered in some cases, but in these forms, disease-modifying treatment is preferred [5].

- Treatment volume per PEX: 1.0–1.5 EPV; in tryptophan-IA: plasma volume 2.0–2.5 liters; regenerative IA: 2.5 EPV.
- Avoid using ACE inhibitors, especially in tryptophan-IA [6].
- Substitution: albumin (PEX), none in IA.
- Interval between sessions: 48 h.
- End of treatment: generally 5–7 sessions of PEX/IA are performed over 14 days.

Acute Disseminated Encephalomyelitis

Definition Acute disseminated encephalomyelitis (ADEM) is a polyfocal autoimmune demyelinating inflammation of the CNS, occurring usually after infection or vaccination though idiopathic ADEM is possible too. Generally it affects children, though ADEM can be detected in adults; the condition has favorable prognosis.

Pathogenesis and pathophysiology Approx. 85% of ADEM cases occur after viral (e.g., HIV, CMV, EBV) and bacterial (e.g., *M. pneumoniae*, *Borrelia burgdorferi*) infections or post-vaccination (e.g., Rabies, tetanus toxoid). Infectious agents cause autoimmune inflammation in genetically predisposed individuals; molecular mimicry may also play an important role in ADEM pathogenesis.

Clinical presentation Symptoms of ADEM occur up to 60 days after previous infection has resolved. Clinically, general symptoms may be present (fever, vomiting, headache), encephalopathy (seizures, coma, irritability, psychosis, confusion), polyfocal neurological deficits (paraparesis, tetraparesis). Specific lesions are detected on MRI. Anti-MOG (myelin oligodendrocyte glycoprotein) antibodies have been described in relapsing ADEM [7].

Treatment of ADEM In the acute phase, symptomatic treatment, antibiotics, and antiviral drugs can be initiated. Once ADEM is suspected, pulse steroids or IVIG (as second choice) should be initiated. Improvement occurs usually within days after treatment initiation [7].

PEX in the treatment of ADEM In steroid/IVIG-resistant cases, PEX can be used as second-line treatment. The procedure is safe in the pediatric population too [8]. The following schedule is recommended [5]:

- Treatment volume per PEX: 1.0–1.5 EPV.
- Substitution: albumin.
- Interval between sessions: 48 h.
- End of treatment: clinical recovery achieved; usually 5–7 sessions are performed.

N-Methyl-D-Aspartate Receptor Antibody (NMDARA) Encephalitis

Definition NMDARA encephalitis is the most common autoimmune encephalitis; it is an autoimmune disease, presenting with IgG autoantibodies against the N-methyl-D-aspartate receptor and specific psychiatric symptoms and motor disturbances [9].

Pathogenesis and pathophysiology NMDARA encephalitis is associated with tumors—most frequently teratomas, but also carcinomas (lung, testicular). Viral infections (herpes simplex virus (HSV)) can also cause NMRD autoantibody production; however, in some cases, etiology remains unclear. The etiologic factor causes autoantibody production against the N-methyl-D-aspartate receptor of the neurons, causing their internalization, decreasing synaptic currents; suppression of NMDA receptor activity causes memory, learning, and behavioral pathology [10].

Clinical presentation Typically, young adults are affected, though the condition can be diagnosed in all age groups. The disease may present with prodromal symptoms (fever, headache, nausea). Generally, six major groups of symptoms are established: psychiatric disorder/cognitive impairment, seizures, movement disorders, speech dysfunction, impaired consciousness, autonomic dysfunction/central hypoventilation. Anti-NMDAR autoantibodies are detected in serum and in cerebrospinal fluid; additionally, specific EEG changes are observed. The diagnosis is based in at least one clinical symptom and the presence of autoantibodies [10].

Treatment of NMDAR encephalitis. Role of PEX First-line treatment includes immunosuppression (steroids/IVIG) and PEX/IA (ASFA category 1). Additionally, tumor resection is performed or acyclovir in HSV-associated cases is used. Failure of first-line treatment within 4 weeks from initiation requires second-line agents (Cyclophosphamide, RTX) [5, 10].

- Treatment volume per PEX: 1.0–1.5 EPV; in tryptophan-IA: plasma volume 2.0–2.5 liters; regenerative IA: 2.5 EPV.
- Avoid using ACE inhibitors, especially in tryptophan-IA.
- Substitution: albumin (PEX), none in IA.
- Interval between sessions: 24–48 h.
- End of treatment: clinical improvement; generally 5–12 sessions of PEX/IA are performed over 7–21 days.

Neuromyelitis Optica Spectrum Disorder (NMOSD)

Definition Neuromyelitis optica spectrum disorder (NMOSD) is a rare autoimmune inflammation, affecting the optical nerve and spinal cord.

Pathogenesis and pathophysiology NMOSD is associated with the presence of Ig G autoantibodies against aquaporin-4. Aquaporin 4 channels are astrocyte transmembrane water channels; their highest density is in the optical nerve, spinal cord, and area postrema. The autoimmune inflammation causes demyelination, affecting predominately the abovementioned areas. The exact etiology of the condition is unknown, but genetic predisposition has been suggested. Associations with other autoimmune diseases have been reported.

Clinical presentation NMOSD encompasses several clinical syndromes [11]:

- Optic neuritis
- Acute myelitis
- Area postrema syndrome (unexplained hiccups, nausea, or vomiting)
- Acute brainstem syndrome
- Symptomatic narcolepsy or acute diencephalic clinical syndrome
- Symptomatic cerebral syndrome
- Imaging: characteristic NMOSD brain/optical nerve lesions on MRI
- Aquaporin-4 IgG autoantibodies: detected in serum, in up to 90% in the patients

Treatment of NMOSD The disease may have a relapsing course, as well as acute monophasic course. Therefore, the treatment of the acute episode is followed by chronic immunosuppressive therapy. Pulse steroids and IVIG are used in the acute attack/relapse. Refractory cases require PEX. Maintenance treatment consists of Azathioprine/RTX/mycophenolate preparations.

Role of PEX in NMOSD PEX, as well as IA, is initiated as second-line therapy in cases of unresponsive to steroids acute attack/relapse (lack of sufficient clinical response from treatment 3 to 5 day after steroid therapy is initiated) (ASFA category 2) [5]. Maintenance PEX/IA may also be beneficial, as, repeated apheresis and/or steroids were found to reduce the number of non-responders to therapy [12].

PEX/IA can be used as first-line treatment in the following situations [12]:

- Insufficient response to glucocorticoids during previous attacks
- Sufficient response to apheresis therapy during previous attacks
- Severe myelitis

The following PEX/IA schedule is recommended [5]:

- Treatment volume per PEX: 1.0–1.5 EPV; in tryptophan-IA: plasma volume 2.0–2.5 liters; regenerative IA: 2.5PV.
- Avoid using ACE inhibitors, especially in tryptophan-IA.
- Substitution: albumin (PEX), none in IA.
- Interval between sessions: 24–48 h.
- End of treatment: clinical improvement; usually 5 sessions of PEX/IA are performed over 10 days; however, up to 10 sessions can be performed.

Diseases of the Peripheral Nervous System

Guillain-Barré Syndrome (GBS)

Definition GBS represents an acute inflammatory disease, affecting the peripheral nervous system. Its clinical presentation includes the typical symptoms of muscle weakness, sensory disturbances, but also autonomic dysfunction, cranial nerve involvement, respiratory failure, and pain [13].

Pathogenesis and pathophysiology The disease is caused by immune inflammation, triggered in approx. 70% of the cases by infection (gastrointestinal, respiratory). Antigen mimicry is the probable pathogenic mechanism, due to the similarity of certain infectious antigens to membrane gangliosides of the peripheral nerves [14]. Several anti-ganglioside antibodies are detected (anti-GD1a, anti-GM1, anti-GC1B), aiming at different nerve targets, thus explaining the multifaceted clinical presentation.

Clinical presentation Classically, GBS presents with acute onset of symmetrical muscle weakness and sensory disturbances. Distal and proximal muscle groups are involved, including neck muscles. Hypo- and areflexia are present. Involvement of autonomic nerves can present with cardiac arrhythmias and blood pressure instability; cranial nerve involvement causes facial diplegia, dysphagia, respiratory muscle weakness, and respiratory disturbances. Subforms of GBS are also present: acute motor axonal neuropathy (motor involvement, without sensory deficits, preserved reflexes); regional sub-types (e.g., pharyngeal–cervical–brachial GBS); Miller-Fisher syndrome (ophthalmoplegia, areflexia, and ataxia) [13]. GBS has monophasic course; relapse or remitting of the disease is atypical.

The diagnosis is based on clinical findings; autoantibody testing also can assist the diagnosis, e.g., in Miller–Fisher syndrome. Imaging is used mainly to differentiate GBS from other neurological issues. Nerve conduction study is also an important part of patient evaluation. Cerebrospinal fluid (CSF) findings consist of an increased CSF protein concentration and a normal WBC count in CSF [13].

Treatment of GBS. Role of PEX PEX or IVIG is a first-line treatment in GBS. Studies have demonstrated that the use of steroids had no clinical benefits [14]. PEX was the first treatment to demonstrate significant improvement in outcomes in GBS patients, making it first-line treatment for the disease (ASFA category 1) [5, 15]. IVIG (400 mg/kg/daily for 5 consecutive days) were found to be equally effective as PEX in GBS. However, a second-line IVIG treatment in GBS patients has no significant benefit but is associated with adverse events; therefore, a second course of IVIG should be avoided in GBS [16]. IA can also be used in GBS and is regarded as first-line treatment. PEX/IA should be performed with caution in autonomic nerve involvement due to hemodynamic instability [5]. The following therapeutic schedule is recommended:

- Treatment volume per PEX: 1.0–1.5 EPV; regenerative IA: up to 3EPV.
- Substitution: albumin (PEX), none in IA.
- Interval between sessions: 24–48 h.
- End of treatment: clinical improvement; usually 5 sessions of PEX/IA are performed over 10 days.

Chronic Inflammatory Demyelinating Polyradiculoneuropathy (CIDP)

Definition CIDP is an autoimmune chronic inflammation of the peripheral nerves, presenting with proximal/distal weakness over >8 weeks; progressive monophasic presentation is more frequently observed, but atypical variants also exist [17].

Pathogenesis and pathophysiology Etiology of the disease is unknown; most of the cases are regarded as idiopathic, though an association with infection (gastrointestinal or respiratory) has been suggested. In CIDP, autoimmune inflammation is the key process, in which humoral (autoantibodies) and cell factors (abnormal macrophage activity) play a pivotal role, leading to demyelination and clinical symptoms [18].

Clinical presentation Six clinical types are defined. Classical CIDP encompasses almost 50% of the cases and presents with progressive or relapsing, symmetric, proximal, and distal muscle weakness of upper and lower limbs and sensory involvement of at least two limbs; development over 8 weeks or more and absent or reduced tendon reflexes in all limbs.

CIDP variants are also observed: Distal CIDP (distal sensory loss and muscle weakness predominantly in lower limbs), multifocal CIDP (multifocal pattern, asymmetric), focal CIDP (only one limb affected), motor CIDP (no sensory involvement), sensory CIDP (no motor involvement).

Diagnosis includes clinical symptoms and nerve conduction studies; testing for nodal and paranodal antibodies can be considered. All patients should be tested for monoclonal paraproteins [19].

Treatment of CIDP. Role of PEX High dose/pulse steroids, IVIG (2 g/kg total dose, over 5 days), and PEX are regarded as first-line therapies in CIDP. As the disease has chronic or relapsing course, maintenance therapy (steroids, IVIG, PEX, RTX, mycophenolate preparations, subcutaneous immunoglobulin, and calcineurin inhibitors) is required. Steroids, IVIG, and PEX are regarded as equally effective treatment options. However, current guidelines weakly recommend IVIG to PEX due to the ease of administration especially in the pediatric population [19]. Yet PEX can be effective when steroids and IVIG fail to control the disease [20].

Tryptophan-IA was also effective in CIDP with similar safety profile to PEX [21]. The following therapeutic schedule is recommended [5]:

- Treatment volume per PEX: 1.0–1.5 EPV; in tryptophan-IA: plasma volume 2.0–2.5 liters.
- Avoid using ACE inhibitors, especially in tryptophan-IA.
- Substitution: albumin (PEX), none in IA.
- Interval between sessions: 2–3 days; usually 2–3 PEX sessions are performed weekly.
- End of treatment: clinical improvement; maintenance treatment 1 PEX per week/1 PEX per month may be considered.

Myasthenia Gravis (MG)

Definition MG is an autoimmune disease, caused by autoantibodies against post-synaptic membrane proteins in the neuromuscular junction, leading to muscle weakness and fatigue of skeletal muscles.

Pathogenesis and pathophysiology The exact etiology of the disease is unknown, but triggering factors like infections, immunizations, surgery, as well as thymoma were identified. In MG, several autoantibodies were detected [22]:

- IgG autoantibodies against nicotinic acetylcholine receptor (nACHR) are present in up to 85% of the cases; anti-nACHR antibodies bind to the nACHR and cause complement-mediated damage, increased nACHR turnover, and loss of nACHR in the post-synaptic membrane, disrupting neuromuscular transmission and causing muscle weakness.

- Antibodies against muscle-specific kinase (MUSK), a tyrosine kinase on the post-synaptic membrane, engaged in the development and maintenance of nACHR clusters on the post-synaptic membrane; anti-MUSK autoantibodies impair MUSK function, finally causing neuromuscular junction dysfunction.
- Antibodies against lipoprotein-related protein 4 (LPRP4). LPRP4 interacts with MUSK and the protein molecule *agrin*, forming MUSK-LPRP4-agrin complex, engaged in formation and maintenance of ACHR clusters.
- Anti-agrin antibodies—least commonly detected, suppressing nACHR cluster formation and maintenance, by suppressing MUSK-LPRP4-agrin complex.

Clinical presentation MG presents with fluctuating muscle weakness, which is more pronounced after physical activity and improves after rest. Typical MG presentation:

- Extraocular muscle weakness (diplopia and ptosis).
- Bulbar muscle weakness (difficulty in chewing, hoarseness, and dysarthria).
- Limb weakness (proximal muscles and upper limbs more frequently affected).
- Myasthenic crisis (involvement of intercostal muscles, diaphragm), risk for respiratory failure, and medical emergency.
- Autonomic nervous system is spared.
- The diagnosis also requires autoantibody testing, nerve conductive studies, and imaging (screening for thymoma) [23]. Seronegative MG may also be diagnosed.

Treatment of MG. Role of PEX Current therapy of MG has significantly improved the outcomes; yet MG crisis is still associated with increased mortality risk.

Generally, treatment of mild exacerbations and maintenance therapy consist of anticholinesterase inhibitors, immunosuppression (steroids, cyclophosphamide, azathioprine, calcineurin inhibitors, RTX, eculizumab). Thymectomy is considered in cases of thymoma.

In MG crisis and refractory/unstable MG, IVIG and PEX are used as first-line therapy, including seronegative MG. Additionally, PEX is effective in stabilizing patients prior to thymectomy [24]. IVIG is easier to apply; however, clinical improvement was observed earlier in PEX, especially in critically ill patients [25]. PEX requires additional immunosuppression. Other apheresis options—IA and double filtration plasmapheresis (DFPP)—are equally effective to PEX; due to their relatively short, lasting effect, PEX/IA/DFPP should be coupled with immunosuppressive therapy [5]. PEX can be performed during pregnancy complicated with MG crisis; patients should be monitored for hypovolemia [26].

The following apheresis schedule in MG is recommended [5]:

- Treatment volume per PEX/DFFP: 1.0–1.5 EPV; tryptophan-IA: plasma volume 2.0–2.5 liters; regenerative IA: 2.5EPV.
- Avoid using ACE inhibitors, especially in tryptophan-IA.
- Substitution: albumin ± FFP (PEX/DFFP), none in IA.
- Interval between sessions: 24–48 h, usually 3–6 procedures in acute MG crisis; initiate immunosuppressive therapy.
- End of treatment: clinical improvement; chronic treatment can be also performed (1 procedure/7–14 days).

Other Neurological Diseases

Lambert Eaton Myasthenic Syndrome (LEMS) LEMS is an autoimmune disease, with antibodies targeting pre-synaptic P/Q type voltage-gated calcium channels of the neuromuscular junction. LEMS is linked to lung cancer and presents with proximal muscle weakness, autonomic dysfunction, and hyporeflexia. Immunosuppression (steroids, IVIG, and cyclophosphamide) and symptomatic treatment (blockers of voltage-gated potassium channels) are usually the first-line treatments. PEX is applied in refractory cases (ASFA category 2). The schedule is similar to MG; the treatment is performed until resolution of symptoms and improvement in nerve conductive tests are established [5].

Voltage-gated potassium channel antibody disorders (VGPCD) VGPCD present clinically with the following syndromes: neuromyotonia, limbic encephalitis, and Morvan syndrome. The disorders are associated with antibodies aiming the voltage-gated potassium channels and may be linked to thymoma, lung cancer, and MG [27]. Treatment consists of immunosuppression (steroids, IVIG, mycophenolate preparations). PEX/IA are used in refractory cases, though they can be used as first-line treatment in certain patients (ASFA category 2). Therapeutic schedule is similar to the one in MG; usually 5–10 procedures are required. Resolution of clinical symptoms is the principal parameter that guides treatment [5].

References

1. Ghasemi N, Razavi S, Nikzad E. Multiple sclerosis: pathogenesis, symptoms, diagnoses and cell-based therapy. Cell J. 2017;19(1):1–10. https://doi.org/10.22074/cellj.2016.4867.
2. Kasper LH, Shoemaker J. Multiple sclerosis immunology: the healthy immune system vs the MS immune system. Neurology. 2010;74(Suppl 1):S2–8. https://doi.org/10.1212/WNL.0b013e3181c97c8f.
3. Ömerhoca S, Yazici Akkaş S, Kale IN. Multiple sclerosis: diagnosis and differential diagnosis. Noropsik Ars. 2018;55(Suppl 1):S1–9. https://doi.org/10.29399/npa.23418.
4. Ramo-Tello C, Blanco Y, Brieva L, Casanova B, Cáceres EM, Ontaneda D, et al. Recommendations for the diagnosis and treatment of multiple sclerosis relapses. J Pers Med. 2022;12(1):6. https://doi.org/10.3390/jpm12010006.
5. Connelly-Smith L, Alquist CR, Aqui NA, Hofmann JC, Klingel R, Onwuemene OA, et al. Guidelines on the use of therapeutic apheresis in clinical practice—evidence-based approach from the writing Committee of the American Society for Apheresis: the ninth special issue. J Clin Apher. 2023;38(2):77–278. https://doi.org/10.1002/jca.22043.
6. Hamilton P, Harris R, Mitra S. Immunoadsorption techniques and its current role in the intensive care unit [Internet]. In: Aspects in continuous

renal replacement therapy. IntechOpen; 2019. Available from: https://doi.org/10.5772/intechopen.84890.

7. Paolilo RB, Deiva K, Neuteboom R, Rostásy K, Lim M. Acute disseminated encephalomyelitis: current perspectives. Children. 2020;7(11):210. https://doi.org/10.3390/children7110210.
8. Savransky A, Rubstein A, Rios MH, Vergel SL, Velasquez MC, Sierra SP, et al. Prognostic indicators of improvement with therapeutic plasma exchange in pediatric demyelination. Neurology. 2019;93(22):e2065–73. https://doi.org/10.1212/WNL.0000000000008551.
9. Dalmau J, Graus F. Antibody-mediated encephalitis. N Engl J Med. 2018;378(9):840–51. https://doi.org/10.1056/NEJMra1708712.
10. Huang Q, Xie Y, Hu Z, Tang X. Anti-N-methyl-D-aspartate receptor encephalitis: a review of pathogenic mechanisms, treatment, prognosis. Brain Res. 2020;1727:146549. https://doi.org/10.1016/j.brainres.2019.146549.
11. Wingerchuk DM, Banwell B, Bennett JL, Cabre P, Carroll W, Chitnis T, et al. International consensus diagnostic criteria for neuromyelitis optica spectrum disorders. Neurology. 2015;85(2):177–89. https://doi.org/10.1212/WNL.0000000000001729.
12. Kümpfel T, Giglhuber K, Aktas O, Ayzenberg I, Bellmann-Strobl J, Häußler V, et al. Update on the diagnosis and treatment of neuromyelitis optica spectrum disorders (NMOSD)—revised recommendations of the Neuromyelitis Optica Study Group (NEMOS). Part II: Attack therapy and long-term management. J Neurol. 2024;271(1):141–76. https://doi.org/10.1007/s00415-023-11910-z.
13. van Doorn PA, Van den Bergh PYK, Hadden RDM, Avau B, Vankrunkelsven P, Attarian S, et al. European Academy of Neurology/Peripheral Nerve Society guideline on diagnosis and treatment of Guillain–Barré syndrome. Eur J Neurol. 2023;30(12):3646–74. https://doi.org/10.1111/ene.16073.
14. Hughes RAC. Guillain-Barré syndrome: history, pathogenesis, treatment, and future directions. Eur J Neurol. 2024;31(11):e16346. https://doi.org/10.1111/ene.16346.
15. Chevret S, Hughes RA, Annane D. Plasma exchange for Guillain-Barré syndrome. Cochrane Database Syst Rev. 2017;2(2):CD001798. https://doi.org/10.1002/14651858.CD001798.pub3.
16. Walgaard C, Jacobs BC, Lingsma HF, Steyerberg EW, Van den Berg B, Doets AY, et al. Second intravenous immunoglobulin dose in patients with Guillain-Barré syndrome with poor prognosis (SID-GBS): a double-blind, randomised, placebo-controlled trial. Lancet Neurol. 2021;20(4):275–83. https://doi.org/10.1016/S1474-4422(20)30494-4.
17. Roman-Guzman RM, Martinez-Mayorga AP, Guzman-Martinez LD. Chronic inflammatory demyelinating polyneuropathy: a narrative review of a systematic diagnostic approach to avoid misdiagnosis. Cureus. 2025;17(1):e76749. https://doi.org/10.7759/cureus.76749.

18. Koike H, Katsuno M. Pathophysiology of chronic inflammatory demyelinating polyneuropathy: insights into classification and therapeutic strategy. Neurol Ther. 2020;9(2):213–27. https://doi.org/10.1007/s40120-020-00190-8.
19. Van den Bergh PYK, van Doorn PA, Hadden RDM, Avau B, Vankrunkelsven P, Allen JA, et al. European Academy of Neurology/Peripheral Nerve Society guideline on diagnosis and treatment of chronic inflammatory demyelinating polyradiculoneuropathy: report of a joint task force—second revision. Eur J Neurol. 2021;28(11):3556–83. https://doi.org/10.1111/ene.14959.
20. Lieker I, Slowinski T, Harms L, Hahn K, Klehmet J. A prospective study comparing tryptophan immunoadsorption with therapeutic plasma exchange for the treatment of chronic inflammatory demyelinating polyneuropathy. J Clin Apher. 2017;32(6):486–93. https://doi.org/10.1002/jca.21546.
21. Kuitwaard K, Hahn AF, Vermeulen M, Venance SL, Van Doorn PA. Intravenous immunoglobulin response in treatmentnaïve chronic inflammatory demyelinating polyradiculoneuropathy. J Neurol Neurosurg Psychiatry. 2015;86(12):1331–6. https://doi.org/10.1136/jnnp-2014-309042.
22. Phillips WD, Vincent A. Pathogenesis of myasthenia gravis: update on disease types, models, and mechanisms. F1000Res. 2016;5:F1000 Faculty Rev-1513. https://doi.org/10.12688/f1000research.8206.1.
23. Rousseff RT. Diagnosis of myasthenia gravis. J Clin Med. 2021;10(8):1736. https://doi.org/10.3390/jcm10081736.
24. Alhaidar MK, Abumurad S, Soliven B, Rezania K. Current treatment of myasthenia gravis. J Clin Med. 2022;11(6):1597. https://doi.org/10.3390/jcm11061597.
25. Rønager J, Ravnborg M, Hermansen I, Vorstrup S. Immunoglobulin treatment versus plasma exchange in patients with chronic moderate to severe myasthenia gravis. Artif Organs. 2001;25(12):967–73. https://doi.org/10.1046/j.1525-1594.2001.06717.x.
26. Bansal R, Goyal MK, Modi M. Management of myasthenia gravis during pregnancy. Indian J Pharmacol. 2018;50(6):302–8. https://doi.org/10.4103/ijp.IJP_452_17.
27. Merchut MP. Management of voltage-gated potassium channel antibody disorders. Neurol Clin. 2010;28(4):941–59. https://doi.org/10.1016/j.ncl.2010.03.024.

Indications for PEX: Endocrinology and Metabolic Disease

7

Abstract

Several metabolic molecules have harmful effect on clinical outcomes. Usually serum levels are controlled by medications. However, in certain clinical scenarios, conservative treatment fails to achieve its therapeutic goals (familial hypercholesterolemia and fulminant Wilson's disease) and direct removal by PEX or other apheresis modalities (e.g. lipoprotein apheresis) may be required. The chapter will review the major indications for PEX in endocrinology and metabolic disease.

Keywords

Familial hypercholesterolemia · Fulminant Wilson disease · Thyroid storm · Lipoprotein apheresis

Familial Hypercholesterolemia

Definition Familial hypercholesterolemia (FH) is an inherited disorder of lipoprotein metabolism, associated with persistently elevated LDL cholesterol and early development of cardiovascular complications. Genetic mutations of the LDL-receptor pathway are mostly inherited in autosomal dominant fashion; patients affected with FH can be homozygous and heterozygous carriers

J. J. Filipov, *Therapeutic Plasma Exchange*, In Clinical Practice,
https://doi.org/10.1007/978-3-032-17275-4_7

of the genetic mutation, which is associated with different outcomes in the two groups [1].

Pathogenesis and pathophysiology Approximately 90% of the patients have mutations of the LDL-receptor gene; other mutations, impairing LDL uptake from LDL receptors, are also detected—apolipoprotein B (ApoB) gene mutation, resulting in decreased binding of LDL to the LDL-receptor, as well as mutations of proprotein convertase subtilisin/kexin 9 (PCSK9) gene, responsible for increased destruction of LDL-receptor. Genetic mutations cause impaired LDL-receptor pathway, disrupting LDL particle endocytosis and further metabolism. This leads to increased serum LDL cholesterol levels that are often refractory to conservative treatment, which relies on LDL-receptor activity [1, 2].

Clinical presentation FH has different manifestations in homozygous (HoFH) and heterozygous (HeFH) types.

- HoFH is observed in homozygous carriers of genetic mutation or compound/double heterozygous carriers of two genetic autosomal-dominant mutations [3]. LDL receptor is practically absent in HoFH patients. HoFH has a prevalence of 1:170000 up to 1:300000. Clinically HoFH presents with elevated LDL levels (usually >500 mg/dL; >13 mmol/L; however, if LDL >370 mg/dL; >9.6 mmol/L HoFH is suspected), skin and tendon xanthomas, and advanced atherosclerotic cardiovascular disease (presenting with angina pectoris in children, systemic atherosclerosis, aortic supravalvular/valvular stenosis); HoFH has very poor prognosos without treatment and is associated with early death (within the first 30 years) [1].
- HeFH has a prevalence of 1:250 worldwide. It is generally asymptomatic. Xanthomas are rare (less than 15%), but their incidence increases with age of untreated cases [2]. LDL is elevated, but less than HoFH (LDL ≥160 mg/dL; ≥4.1 mmol/L for children, LDL ≥190 mg/dL; ≥4.9 mmol/L for adults). Diagnosis often requires genetic testing, as well as family history for premature coronary artery disease, xanthomas, and hypercholesterolemia [2, 4].

Treatment of FH Conservative treatment should be initiated as early as possible, especially for HoFH. Lipid lowering treatment, as well as diet modification, life style changes are required. Treatment of accompanying conditions (hypertension, diabetes mellitus) should be performed.

Medical treatment includes the following groups of drugs: statins, ezetimibe, bile acid sequestrants (colesevelam), and PCSK9 inhibition with human monoclonal antibodies (alirocumab, evolocumab). Microsomal triglyceride transfer protein (MTP) inhibitors (Lomitapide) are a group of drugs that lower LDL independently of the LDL receptor. They are indicated currently only for HoFH and achieve up to 50% reduction of LDL levels [1, 2].

Role of Lipoprotein apheresis and PEX in the treatment of FH Lipoprotein apheresis (LA) plays a pivotal role in the treatment of HoFH (ASFA category 1), alongside with the abovementioned medications, as it eliminates LDL molecules. It is also used in refractory cases in HeFH (ASFA category 2). Though PEX can also be used in FH, it is reserved for situations, where LA is not available or in small children [5].

Generally, a single LA session reduces pre-treatment LDL levels with 50–80%. Different types of LA are available (for more details see section "Lipoprotein Apheresis" of the book, Chap. 2):

- Immunoadsorption—LDL removal is based on the antigen-antibody reaction. Plasma flows through columns, containing antibodies against apolipoprotein B100 (apolB100), which is the plasma protein carrier of LDL molecule. LDL/ApolB100 complexes bind to the antibodies, whereas LDL-free plasma is returned to the patient. LDL IA requires 3–6 liters processed blood for each treatment, achieving up to 40% reduction from pre-treatment LDL levels. The procedure is relatively safe but has a high cost. Additionally, the use of ACE inhibitors in this type of LA is contraindicated, due to the risk for bradykinin accumulation.

- Heparin-induced extracorporeal LDL precipitation (HELP)—Based on the principle of DFPP, LDL molecules are removed by precipitation after being treated with acidic solution of heparin. Initially, plasma is separated from blood; at the second stage, plasma is being processed with acidic solution of heparin; at the third stage, plasma runs through a second filter, removing LDL-heparin precipitates; at the fourth stage, heparin is removed by heparin adsorber. Finally, plasma undergoes bicarbonate dialysis, restoring physiological pH, and is returned to the patient. The procedure achieves up to 50% reduction of pre-treatment LDL levels. As a significant fibrinogen depletion is present, treatment volume is limited to 3 l. In HELP, the use of ACE inhibitors is not contraindicated.
- Double filtration lipid apheresis—The method is again based on DFPP, with a second filter used for the removal of lipoproteins, LDL molecules, and triglycerides. Usually rheofilters are used, which improve microcirculation by effectively removing LDL, VLDL, triglyceride molecules, but also fibrinogen and IgM. The method achieved similar effectiveness (70% LDL reduction) to the HELP technique. Yet, it is far more simplified, compared to HELP. The plasma volume required for the procedure varies between 2500 and 3500 ml. Additionally, DFPP with high permeability plasma component separators, that remove selectively LDL molecules, can be used for lipoprotein apheresis.
- Dextran sulfate-based lipoprotein apheresis—The process resembles IA. After initial separation from blood cells, plasma flows through columns, consisting of cellulose-dextran sulfate. Dextran sulfate is negatively charged and binds to positively charged apolipoprotein B100, carrying LDL molecules; after saturation of the column, rinsing and regeneration are performed. The procedure achieves up to 80% LDL reduction, but a drop in fibrinogen and factor VIII is also present. ACE inhibitors can also cause hypotension by increasing bradykinin levels during dextran sulfate-based LDL apheresis. The use of regenerative columns enables the use of higher treatment volumes (up to 6 liters) [6].

- Direct adsorption of lipoproteins (DALI)—Based on the principles of hemoperfusion, blood runs directly through adsorber, covered with negatively charged polyacrylate molecules. They bind to the positively charged apolipoproteins, thus removing LDL and VLDL. Usually 1.5–2 blood volumes are being processed, resulting in LDL reduction by 60%. A recent study demonstrated that DALI method is inferior to double filtration lipid apheresis [7]. Additionally, ACE inhibitors can cause bradykinin accumulation in DALI.

Lipid apheresis is performed safely and effectively in pregnant women and in children [8, 9].

The following therapeutic scheme is recommended [5, 10]:

- Treatment volume: 1.0–1.5 EPV for PEX; treatment volumes for LA varies according to type of LA.
- ACE inhibitors should be avoided in most of the LA systems (see the abovementioned characteristics of different types of LA).
- Substitution: albumin (PEX), none in LA.
- Vascular access: peripheral veins are usually preferred; peripheral vein access is challenging in small children. Other options for long-term apheresis can also be considered [e.g., arteriovenous fistula (AVF), tunneled central venous catheter]. High rate of AVF failure is present in LA, reaching up to 37% [11].
- Interval between sessions: preferably 7 days (1 LA per week); shorter intervals (2 LA sessions per week) can be performed only in exceptional situations (e.g., pregnancy); in cases of limited access to LA, longer intervals (up to 14 days) between LA sessions can also be considered.
- End of treatment: achievement of target LDL level of ≤120 mg/dl (3.1 mmol/L); chronic treatment in HoHF is required (1 LA per 7–14 days). Constant value for post-apheresis LDL is established after 4 cycles of LA.

Thyroid Storm

Definition Thyroid storm is a severe clinical form of thyrotoxicosis. Its manifestations is triggered by various factors: infection, childbirth, surgery, abrupt discontinuation of anti-thyroid medications, amiodarone treatment. It presents with undetectable thyroid-stimulating hormone (TSH) levels, high triiodothyronine (T3) and thyroxine (T4) levels, and end-organ damage [12].

Pathophysiology Several pathogenic mechanisms are involved in the development of thyroid storm [13]:

- Acute increase of T3 and T4 release
- Acute illness, causing acute decrease in hormone protein binding, leading to elevated free T3 and T4 levels
- Sympathetic nervous system activation
- Increased cellular response to T3/T4 signaling (hypoxemia, infection, lactic acidosis, and ketoacidosis)

Clinical presentation Clinical symptoms include fever >38.0 °C, central nervous system involvement (agitation, delirium, psychosis, seizures), gastrointestinal manifestations (diarrhea, vomiting, abdominal pain), cardiac symptoms [tachycardia (heart rate >130 beats/min), congestive heart failure]. Laboratory findings include elevated free T4/T3 and low TSH levels [12].

Treatment of thyroid storm First-line treatment usually includes several medications: anti-thyroid drugs, steroids, cholestyramine, iodine, β-blockers.

Role of PEX PEX is used in refractory to medical treatment patients. Most typical indications for PEX in thyroid storm are [5, 12]:

- Failure to achieve clinical improvement with first-line treatment within 24–28 h from initiation
- Severe symptoms and rapid clinical deterioration

- Contraindications to medical treatment
- Amiodarone-induced thyrotoxicosis (long T ½ of amiodarone)
- Bridging therapy to thyroidectomy

The following treatment schedule is recommended [5, 14]:

- Treatment volume: 1.0–1.5 EPV.
- Substitution: albumin or FFP.
- Interval between sessions: 24–72 h.
- End of treatment: clinical improvement. Usually 2–6 PEX procedures are required.

Fulminant Wilson Disease

Definition Wilson disease (WD) is a rare autosomal recessive genetic disorder, which is associated with copper accumulation in various organs, most specifically liver, brain, cornea. It may present with hepatic manifestations, neurological and psychiatric symptoms, or combination of these. Fulminant Wilson disease presents with acute liver failure, hemolytic anemia, and multiorgan failure [15].

Pathophysiology In WD, a mutation of adenosine triphosphatase copper transporting beta (*ATP7B*), encoding a metal-transporting P-type adenosine triphosphatase, is detected. The enzyme is predominantly expressed in liver and controls copper excretion into the bile ducts, as well as incorporation of copper in ceruloplasmin. Gene mutation causes decreased copper biliary excretion, leading to hepatocyte copper accumulation; additionally, copper-deficient ceruloplasmin is secreted in the blood, which has shorter half-life and is more rapidly metabolized than copper-containing ceruloplasmin. Toxic copper liver accumulation occurs; once hepatic storage limit is exceeded, hepatic copper is released in blood and is accumulated in other organs (central nervous system, heart, kidneys, cornea, etc.) [15, 16].

Clinical presentation Several clinical patterns of WD are present [15]:

- Hepatic involvement—asymptomatic hepatomegaly; persistently elevated AsAT and AlAT; acute hepatitis, varying severity including acute liver injury; cirrhosis—compensated or decompensated; acute liver failure.
- Neurological involvement—dysarthria; movement disorders, pseudobulbar palsy; transfer dysphagia; rigid dystonia; dysautonomia; seizures; sleep disorders, insomnia.
- Psychiatric involvement—depression, bipolar disorders, neurotic behavior, personality change, psychosis.
- Other organs—eye involvement (Kayser–Fleischer rings and sunflower cataracts); hematologic (non-immune hemolytic anemia); kidneys (Fanconi syndrome, nephrolithiasis, hypouricemia); skeletal abnormalities (osteoporosis, arthritis); heart (cardiomyopathy, arrhythmias); endocrine pathology (hypothyroidism, infertility) and pancreatitis.
- Fulminant WD presents with acute liver failure; hemolytic anemia; coagulopathy, not improving on intravenous vitamin K; rapid deterioration of kidney function; modest rise of AsAT and AlAT.
- Specific laboratory tests: decreased serum ceruloplasmin, elevated ceruloplasmin unbound serum copper levels; increased urine copper excretion; liver biopsy with hepatic parenchymal copper concentration.
- Imaging—brain MRI or CT scan.
- Genetic tests are also available.

Management of WD and fulminant WD. Role of PEX Chelating agents are currently used for the treatment of WD (D-Penicillamine, Trientine, Tetrathiomolybdate) as well as medications reducing intestinal copper uptake (zinc salts). Treatment is initiated even in asymptomatic cases. Additionally, low-copper content in food is required.

In fulminant WD, liver transplantation is required. However, due to the limited donor numbers, supportive measures should be undertaken—chelating agents (if kidney function preserved), zinc salts, and PEX. PEX effectively removes copper from circulation (ASFA category 1 in fulminant WD); substitution with FFP corrects liver-associated coagulopathy. Alternatively, albumin only substitution will worsen present coagulopathy. However, other methods [albumin dialysis, molecular absorbance recirculating system (MARS), hemodialysis/hemofiltration] may be used. These interventions, however, are bridge to liver transplantation; in less than 10% of fulminant WD, liver transplant may not be required [15]. However, a study demonstrated 46% survival rate without liver transplantation in fulminant WD cases, treated with PEX. The following therapeutic scheme is recommended [5]:

- Treatment volume: 1.0–1.5 EPV. High volume PEX (treatment volume >1.5PV) is also possible [17].
- Substitution: FFP or FFP + albumin; do not use albumin-only substitution.
- Interval between sessions: 24–48 h.
- End of treatment: clinical improvement.

Hyperlipidemic (Hypertriglyceridemic) Acute Pancreatitis (HLAP)

Definition Hypertriglyceridemia is a major cause for acute pancreatitis, with incidence ranging from 2% to 4%. Acute pancreatitis usually develops in triglyceride levels >1000 mg/dL (11.3 mmol/L).

Pathogenesis and pathophysiology Though the exact mechanisms for pancreatic injury are not elucidated, several pathways have been suggested: excessive production of fatty acids from extremely elevated triglyceride levels, which pancreatic cell injury and ischemia; hypertriglyceridemia-associated hyperviscosity in pancreatic capillaries, causing pancreatic ischemia. Genetic predisposition cannot be ruled out [18].

Clinical presentation HLAP presents with the typical manifestations of acute pancreatitis: abdominal pain; elevated amylase/lipase more than three times upper limit of normal values; imaging, demonstrating pancreatic findings for acute inflammation. HLAP tends to be more severe than non-HLAP and higher triglyceride levels are associated with higher complication rates and higher risk for organ failure and overall mortality [19].

Treatment of HLAP. Role of PEX The major aspects in the treatment of HLAP are management of acute pancreatitis (aggressive intravenous hydration, bowel rest, and pain control) and triglyceride level reduction (specific for HLAP). Triglyceride reduction includes diet restriction, heparin and insulin infusions. Maintenance therapy should include lipid-lowering medications: fibrates, statins, niacin, and omega three fatty acids [18].

Several blood purification methods are used in HLAP.

Therapeutic apheresis (PEX and LA) may achieve more rapid reduction of triglyceride levels compared to conservative treatment; however, they failed to demonstrate significant improvement in mortality, compared to conservative treatment as well as local and systemic complications [20, 21]. Moreover, a recent study demonstrated higher need for intensive care admission in patients with HLAP, treated with PEX [22]. Possible indications for PEX/LA use in HLAP are [20, 23]:

(a) Serum triglyceride levels are not reduced ˂11.3 mmol/L (1000 mg/dl) or do not decrease by less than 50% or remain elevated after receiving conventional lipid-lowering treatment with heparin, insulin, and lipid-lowering drugs up to 24–48 h of admission.
(b) Patients with persistent organ failure and systemic inflammatory response syndrome (SIRS), despite triglyceride reduction ˂11.3 mmol/L (1000 mg/dl).
(c) Treatment of elevated triglyceride levels without acute pancreatitis in pregnant women to avoid drug toxicity.

Combined purification [PEX/hemoadsorption + continuous veno-venous hemofiltration(CVVH)} was also described; however, further studies are needed to evaluate its benefit in HLAP; in cases where PEX and other apheresis modalities are not available, CVVH only can be used, especially in severe acute pancreatitis [18]. Generally, the indications listed in points "a" and "b" can be used for combined purification too. The following therapeutic scheme is suggested [5, 18]:

- Treatment volume: 1.0–1.5 EPV for PEX; treatment volumes for LA vary according to type of LA.
- ACE inhibitors should be avoided in most of the LA systems.
- Citrate anticoagulation may have benefit over heparin in reducing mortality.
- Substitution: albumin or FFP (PEX), none in LA.
- Interval between sessions: 24 h, 1–3 procedures.
- End of treatment: clinical improvement, reduction in serum triglyceride ˂500 mg/dL (5.6 mmol/L).

References

1. Nohara A, Tada H, Ogura M, Okazaki S, Ono K, Shimano H, et al. Homozygous familial hypercholesterolemia. J Atheroscler Thromb. 2021;28(7):665–78. https://doi.org/10.5551/jat.RV17050.
2. McGowan MP, Hosseini Dehkordi SH, Moriarty PM, Duell PB. Diagnosis and treatment of heterozygous familial hypercholesterolemia. J Am Heart Assoc. 2019;8(24):e013225. https://doi.org/10.1161/JAHA.119.013225.
3. Han Y, Zhang L, Tao H, Wu J, Zhai J. Genetic analysis and management of a familial hypercholesterolemia pedigree with polygenic variants: case report. Medicine (Baltimore). 2023;102(32):e34534. https://doi.org/10.1097/MD.0000000000034534.
4. Gidding SS, Champagne MA, De Ferranti SD, Defesche J, Ito MK, Knowles JW, et al. The agenda for familial hypercholesterolemia: a scientific statement from the American Heart Association. Circulation. 2015;132(22):2167–92.https://doi.org/10.1161/CIR.0000000000000297.
5. Connelly-Smith L, Alquist CR, Aqui NA, Hofmann JC, Klingel R, Onwuemene OA, et al. Guidelines on the use of therapeutic apheresis in clinical practice – evidence-based approach from the writing Committee of the American Society for Apheresis: the ninth special issue. J Clin Apher. 2023;38(2):77–278. https://doi.org/10.1002/jca.22043.

6. Bambauer R, Latza R, Schiel R. Methods. In: Therapeutic plasma exchange and selective plasma separation methods: fundamental technologies, pathophysiology, and clinical results. 4th ed. Frankfurt: Pabst Science Publ; 2013. p. 51–191.
7. Özdemir ZN, Şahin U, Yıldırım Y, Kaya CT, İlhan O. Lipoprotein apheresis efficacy and challenges: single center experience. Hematol Transfus Cell Ther. 2022;44(1):56–62. https://doi.org/10.1016/j.htct.2021.01.009.
8. Lewek J, Bielecka-Dabrowa A, Toth PP, Banach M. Dyslipidaemia management in pregnant patients: a 2024 update. Eur Hear J Open. 2024;4(3):oeae032. https://doi.org/10.1093/ehjopen/oeae032.
9. Taylan C, Driemeyer J, Schmitt CP, Pape L, Büscher R, Galiano M, et al. Cardiovascular outcome of pediatric patients with bi-allelic (homozygous) familial hypercholesterolemia before and after initiation of multimodal lipid lowering therapy including lipoprotein apheresis. Am J Cardiol. 2020;136:38–48. https://doi.org/10.1016/j.amjcard.2020.09.015.
10. France M, Rees A, Datta D, Thompson G, Capps N, Ferns G, et al. HEART UK statement on the management of homozygous familial hypercholesterolaemia in the United Kingdom. Atherosclerosis. 2016;255:128–39. https://doi.org/10.1016/j.atherosclerosis.2016.10.017.
11. Doherty DJ, Pottle A, Malietzis G, Hakim N, Barbir M, Crane JS. Vascular access in lipoprotein apheresis: a retrospective analysis from the UK'S largest lipoprotein apheresis centre. J Vasc Access. 2018;19(1):52–7. https://doi.org/10.5301/jva.5000755.
12. De Almeida R, McCalmon S, Cabandugama PK. Clinical review and update on the management of thyroid storm. Mo Med. 2022;119(4):366–71. PMID: 36118802.
13. Pandey R, Kumar S, Kotwal N. Thyroid storm: clinical manifestation, pathophysiology, and treatment [internet]. In: Goiter - causes and treatment. IntechOpen; 2020. Available from: https://doi.org/10.5772/intechopen.89620.
14. Shinohara M, Uchida T, Funayama T, Watanabe M, Kusaoi M, Yamaji K, et al. Effect of plasma exchange in thyroid storm with consideration of its distribution into the extravascular space. J Endocr Soc. 2020;4(4):bvaa023. https://doi.org/10.1210/jendso/bvaa023.
15. Schilsky ML, Roberts EA, Bronstein JM, Dhawan A, Hamilton JP, Rivard AM, et al. A multidisciplinary approach to the diagnosis and management of wilson disease: 2022 practice guidance on Wilson disease from the American Association for the Study of Liver Diseases. Hepatology. 2025;82(3):E41–90. https://doi.org/10.1002/hep.32801.
16. Patil M, Sheth KA, Krishnamurthy AC, Devarbhavi H. A review and current perspective on Wilson disease. J Clin Exp Hepatol. 2013;3(4):321–36. https://doi.org/10.1016/j.jceh.2013.06.002.
17. Pawaria A, Sood V, Lal BB, Khanna R, Bajpai M, Alam S. Ninety days transplant free survival with high volume plasma exchange in Wilson dis-

ease presenting as acute liver failure. J Clin Apher. 2021;36(1):109–17. https://doi.org/10.1002/jca.21848.
18. Garg R, Rustagi T. Management of hypertriglyceridemia induced acute pancreatitis. Biomed Res Int. 2018;2018:4721357. https://doi.org/10.1155/2018/4721357.
19. Deng LH, Xue P, Xia Q, Yang XN, Wan MH. Effect of admission hypertriglyceridemia on the episodes of severe acute pancreatitis. World J Gastroenterol. 2008;14(28):4558–61. https://doi.org/10.3748/wjg.14.4558.
20. Gubensek J. The role of apheresis and insulin therapy in hypertriglyceridemic acute pancreatitis—a concise review. BMC Gastroenterol. 2023;23(1):341. https://doi.org/10.1186/s12876-023-02957-3.
21. Zheng C, Zheng Y, Zheng Z. Therapeutic plasma exchange decreases serum triglyceride level rapidly and reduces early recurrence rate but no advantages in improving outcomes for patients with hyperlipidemic acute pancreatitis: a retrospective propensity score matching analysis based on twenty year's experience. BMC Endocr Disord. 2024;23(1):341. https://doi.org/10.1186/s12876-023-02957-3.
22. Cao L, Chen Y, Liu S, Huang W, Wu D, Hong D, et al. Early plasmapheresis among patients with hypertriglyceridemia-associated acute pancreatitis. JAMA Netw Open. 2023;6(6):e2320802. https://doi.org/10.1001/jamanetworkopen.2023.20802.
23. Wang J, Xia Y, Cao Y, Cai X, Jiang S, Liao Y, et al. Evaluating the efficacy and timing of blood purification modalities in early-stage hyperlipidemic acute pancreatitis treatment. Lipids Health Dis. 2023;22(1):208. https://doi.org/10.1186/s12944-023-01968-z.

8 Indications for PEX: Cardiology and Pulmonology

Abstract

Plasma exchange (PEX) is used in cardiology for the treatment of idiopathic dilated cardiomyopathy and complications in heart transplantation. Other therapeutic apheresis modalities are also performed in these cases: immunoadsorption (IA) and extracorporeal photopheresis (ECP). Additionally, lipoprotein apheresis is used in the treatment of peripheral artery disease. PEX and ECP are used in the treatment and prevention of lung transplant complications.

Keywords

Idiopathic dilated cardiomyopathy · Heart transplantation · Lung transplantation · Peripheral artery disease · Lipoprotein apheresis

Idiopathic Dilated Cardiomyopathy

Definition Idiopathic dilated cardiomyopathy (IDCM) is a heart muscle disease characterized by left ventricular dilatation and global or regional systolic dysfunction, not associated with cardiac diseases (hypertension, valvular, or congenital heart disease) or coronary artery disease. Its prevalence ranges from 1:250 to

J. J. Filipov, *Therapeutic Plasma Exchange*, In Clinical Practice,
https://doi.org/10.1007/978-3-032-17275-4_8

1:400 individuals in the general population; most of the cases are caused by familial IDCM [1].

Pathogenesis and Pathophysiology Several factors, triggering IDCM, have been evaluated—genetic variants, virus-mediated damage, immune mechanisms, as well as toxic and tachycardia-induced heart muscle damage. Genetic abnormalities are of particular concern due to the high percentage of familial IDCM. Genetic mutations are inherited usually in autosomal dominant fashion, though other inheritance patterns have been described. Additionally, virus infections also cause cardiac damage, probably by triggering autoimmune response (e.g., β1-adrenoreceptor autoantibody) [2].

Clinical Presentation Generally, the patients present with the typical manifestations of left ventricular dysfunction—nocturnal dyspnea, orthopnea, peripheral edema, arrhythmias, and sudden cardiac death. Venous congestion and cardiomegaly are detected on chest X-ray. Exclusion of primary causes for heart failure is required; genetic testing may also be performed. Usually, patients with IDCM tend to be younger (age between 20–60 years, though other age groups may not be spared). Hypothyroidism, anemia, and hemochromatosis should be ruled out. Current guidelines recommend also transthoracic echocardiography and cardiac magnetic resonance [1].

Treatment of IDCM Conservative treatment is the first-line management in IDCM—loop diuretics, ACE inhibitors or angiotensin receptor blockers (ARB), aldosterone receptor blockers, beta-blockers, and anticoagulant medications; steroids and intravenous immunoglobulin can be used. Additionally, in resynchronization therapy, use of implanted cardioverter defibrillator and heart transplantation may be considered in advanced IDCM [2].

Role of PEX and IA in IDCM Immunoadsorption has been studied more extensively in ICDM. IA was found to improve clinical symptoms and ejection fraction; the improvement is particularly detected in cases of high cardiac autoantibody titers [3]. PEX is performed in cases when IA is not available and in pediatric patients, as PEX requires lower extracorporeal volumes.

The following therapeutic regimen is suggested [4]:

- Treatment volume per PEX: 1.0–1.5 plasma volumes (PV); in tryptophan-IA: plasma volume 2.0–2.5 L; regenerative IA: 2.5PV.
- Do not use ACE inhibitors, especially in tryptophan-IA.
- Substitution: albumin (PEX), none in IA.
- Interval between sessions: 24–48 h.
- End of treatment: clinical improvement; usually five sessions of PEX/IA are required; maintenance treatment may also be performed.

Heart Transplantation: Desensitization

Definition AB0 incompatibility and pre-transplant donor-specific HLA—antibodies are significant obstacle to heart transplantation (HT); they are associated with a lower likelihood of heart transplantation and poorer post-transplant outcomes [5].

Pathogenesis, Pathophysiology, Clinical Importance The presence of isohemagglutinins (AB0 incompatible HT) and donor-specific anti-HLA- antibodies (DSA-HLA) prior to HT may predispose to acute antibody-mediated rejection (AbMR) in the post-transplant period. Therefore, specific measures, including immunosuppression and plasma exchange, may be required in the pre-transplant setting [5].

Management of Sensitized HT Candidates. Role of PEX

In AB0i HT with donor-specific isohemagglutinin titer >1:8, pre-transplant PEX should be considered. In cases with isohemagglutinin titer lower than 1:4 PEX may not be necessary. In cases with titers higher than 1:16, modification of immunosuppressive treatment may be needed too. Isohemagglutinin titer >1:8 requires anti-thymocyte globulin (ATG) induction; titer >1:32 requires the use of Rituximab perioperatively and may be added post-transplant in rising isohemagglutinin titers. Generally, standard maintenance immunosuppression, similar to AB0 compatible HT, is used. It should be noted that strategies for the pediatric population may differ from the adult patients [6].

Presence of DSA-HLA is an obstacle to successful HT. Previously elevated panel reactive antibodies (PRA) ≥ 10% was associated with higher risk for acute rejection and mortality post-HT, current guidelines support desensitization initiation at calculated PRA > 50%; thresholds for mean fluorescence intensity (MFI) vary between centers, though MFI<5000 is usually regarded as acceptable rejection risk [6, 7]. Desensitization includes intravenous immunoglobulin (IVIG) and PEX, either alone or in combination; despite its effectiveness, the treatment is associated with DSA-HLA rebound [7]. Therefore, additional therapies can be added, improving effectiveness and reducing the risk for rebound (e.g., Rituximab and Bortezomib), limiting the use of PEX as monotherapy [4, 5]. IA can also be used in pre-HT desensitization.

The following PEX regimen is suggested:

- Treatment volume per PEX: 1.0–1.5 EPV.
- Substitution: albumin, FFP.
- Interval between sessions: 24–48 h.
- End of treatment: negative isohemagglutinin levels; undetectable DSA-HLA. Post-transplant PEX sessions may be performed.

Heart Transplantation: Acute Rejection

Definition Acute rejection (AR) post-HT is inflammatory response directed at myocytes/capillaries of the graft. There are two types of acute rejection: cellular AR (ACR) and acute antibody-mediated (AbMR). Risk factors for acute rejection are young age of heart transplant recipient, female recipient/donor, HLA sensitization, higher HLA mismatches. Endomyocardial biopsy is the golden standard for ACR and AbMR diagnosis.

Pathophysiology and Histological Findings

- In ACR, activated antigen-presenting cells migrate to secondary lymphoid tissue; they present donor peptides to CD8+/CD4+ T cells, triggering the activation of alloreactive T-effectors; CD8+ T-cells produce cytokines and cause direct graft injury. CD4+ T helpers type 1 and macrophages cause delayed hypersensitivity and inflammation. ACR is characterized with lymphocyte and macrophage infiltration, causing myocyte damage. In severe cases, edema hemorrhage and vasculitis are present [8].
- In AbMR, the activated antigen presenting cells present the antigens to CD4+ T cells, which activate B cells; thus, the formation of plasma cells and synthesis of DSA-HLA-Ab is initiated. The antibodies bind to the antigen and activate complement cascade, leading to cellular death. Histologically interstitial edema, hemorrhage, and neutrophilic infiltration in and around capillaries are detected; positive staining for CD68 and C4d is also present [9].

Clinical Presentation ACR post-HT presents with different aspects of heart failure: orthopnea, shortness of breath, peripheral edema; persistent ventricular/atrial tachyarrhythmias also require evaluation for rejection. The golden standard for rejection diagnosis is endomyocardial biopsy and testing for DSA-HLA-Ab [8].

Management of Acute Rejection. Role of PEX and Extracorporeal Photopheresis (ECP)

- Acute cellular rejection: High dose steroids are the first-line treatment of ACR after HT. If clinical improvement is not detected within 12–24 h, ATG is added to the treatment. Additionally, correction of maintenance immunosuppression is required. In recurrent/resistant ACR, after these measures have been applied, the use of extracorporeal photopheresis (ECP) or total lymphoid irradiation may be performed [6].
- Acute AbMR: The following medications—high-dose steroids, ATG, Rituximab, Bortezomib, Eculizumab. Additionally, PEX or immunoadsorption (IA) coupled with IVIG can be used. IA is more specific, but less effective in removing DSA-HLA-Ab, compared to PEX; it is associated with better hemodynamic stability [6].

Therapeutic schedule for ECP [4]:

- Two types of ECP are present: in-line ECP, in which UVA radiation occurs during the centrifugation of leukocytes, and off-line ECP, in which WBC separation on UV radiation occurs in different devices, so the patient is disconnected from the separation device once WBC separation is accomplished. In-line ECP processes 1.5 L of blood; in off-line ECP, larger blood volumes are processed (3.5–10 L). Two procedures in two consecutive days are regarded as one cycle.
- Treatment volume per procedure (whole blood): 1.5 L (in-line ECP); 3–10 L (off-line ECP).
- Substitution: none.
- Frequency of treatment cycles: initially 1 treatment cycle per week, gradually reduced to 1 cycle over 6 weeks.
- End of treatment: clinical improvement.

Therapeutic schedule for PEX [4, 6]:

- Treatment volume: 1.0–1.5 EPV.
- Substitution: albumin, FFP.
- Interval between procedures: 24–48 h over 5 days; less intensive regimens (1 PEX per week over 2–4 weeks) are also possible.
- End of treatment: clinical improvement.

Peripheral Artery Disease

Definition Peripheral artery disease (PAD) is an atherosclerotic disorder, associated with stenosis or occlusion of large and medium-size arteries (excluding coronary and cerebrovascular arteries), and a highly prevalent condition, which is associated with high mortality risk. However, due to its asymptomatic course, in more than 50% of the patients, it is widely underdiagnosed [10].

Risk Factors, Clinical Presentation Generally, the risk factors for PAD are well established: diabetes mellitus, smoking, age, and race. PAD is asymptomatic in most of the cases; symptomatic PAD most frequently affects femoral and popliteal arteries. Clinically, PAD may present with effort-induced claudication, as well as chronic ischemia, presenting with ischemic rest pain and ulceration/gangrene; different diagnostic tools have been suggested to enhance the diagnosis of PAD (e.g., measurement of ankle-brachial index, duplex ultrasound, CT angiography) [11].

Management of PAD The first-line treatment in PAD is lifestyle change, diabetes control, correction of dyslipidemia, blood pressure control anti-thrombotic therapy. In severe PAD, surgical/endovascular revascularization may be required.

Role of Lipoprotein Apheresis (LA) In LA LDL molecules, lipoproteins and fibrinogen are removed, which can lead to improved clinical outcomes in PAD (improved ankle-brachial index, decreased cardiovascular, and cerebrovascular events). A recent study demonstrated improved clinical outcomes from LA in PAD patients with controlled dyslipidemia, indicating that its beneficial effect spans beyond lipid molecule removal [12, 13].

Different types of LA are available (for more details see section "Lipoprotein Apheresis" of the book):

- Immunoadsorption: LDL removal is based on the antigen-antibody reaction. Plasma flows through columns, containing antibodies against apolipoprotein B100 (apolB100), which is the plasma protein carrier of LDL molecule. LDL/ApolB100 complexes bind to the antibodies, whereas LDL-free plasma is returned to the patient. LDL IA requires 3–6 L processed blood for each treatment. The procedure is relatively safe but has a high cost. Additionally, the use of ACE inhibitors in this type of LA is contraindicated, due to the risk for bradykinin accumulation.
- Heparin-induced extracorporeal LDL precipitation (HELP): based on the principle of double filtration plasmapheresis (DFPP), LDL molecules are removed by precipitation after being treated with acidic solution of heparin. Initially, plasma is separated from blood; at the second stage, plasma is being processed with acidic solution of heparin; at the third stage, plasma runs through a second filter, removing LDL-heparin precipitates; at the fourth stage, heparin is removed by heparin adsorber. Finally, plasma undergoes bicarbonate dialysis, restoring physiological pH, and is returned to the patient. As a significant fibrinogen depletion is present, treatment volume is limited to 3 l. In HELP, the use of ACE inhibitors is not contraindicated.
- Double filtration lipid apheresis: The method is again based on DFPP, with a second filter used for removal of lipoproteins, LDL molecules, and triglycerides. Usually, rheofilters are used, which improve microcirculation by effectively removing LDL, VLDL, triglyceride molecules, but also fibrinogen and IgM. The plasma volume required for the procedure varies between 2500 and 3500 ml.DFPP, using high permeability

plasma component separators selectively removes LDL molecules too.

- Dextran sulfate-based Lipoprotein apheresis: The process resembles IA. After initial separation from blood cells, plasma flows through columns, consisting of cellulose-dextran sulfate. Dextran sulfate is negatively charged and binds to positively charged apolipoprotein B100, carrying LDL molecules; after saturation of the column, rinsing and regeneration is performed. The procedure achieves up to 80% LDL reduction, but a drop in fibrinogen and factor VIII is also present. ACE inhibitors cause hypotension by increasing bradykinin levels during dextran sulfate-based lipoprotein apheresis. The use of regenerative columns enables the use of higher treatment volumes (up to 6 L).
- Direct adsorption of lipoproteins (DALI): Based on the principles of hemoperfusion, blood runs directly through adsorber, covered with negatively charged polyacrylate molecules. They bind to the positively charged apolipoproteins, thus removing LDL and VLDL. Usually 1.5–2 blood volumes are being processed. ACE inhibitors can cause bradykinin accumulation in DALI.

The following treatment schedules are suggested [4, 13]:

- Treatment volume: treatment volumes for LA varies according to type of LA.
- ACE inhibitors should be avoided in most of the LA systems (see the above-mentioned characteristics of different types of LA).
- Substitution: none in LA.
- Interval between LA 1–2 sessions per week (short treatment), chronic treatment 14 days per LA.
- End of treatment: usually 5 to 10 procedures are performed; longer treatment can be considered.

Lung Transplantation

Desensitization in Lung Transplantation The presence of pre-transplant DSA-HLA Ab is associated with higher risk for AbMR and poorer survival in lung transplant recipients [14]. According to the Toronto lung transplant HLA antibody protocol, lung transplant candidates with PRA >30% and high urgency candidates are short-listed for desensitization [15]. A recent paper by the same team demonstrated similar clinical post-transplant outcomes in lung transplantation, after desensitization with PEX (first procedure performed intraoperatively), IVIG, and ATG [16].

The following desensitization is suggested by the Toronto lung transplant HLA antibody protocol [15, 16]:

- Treatment volume: 3EPV—initial intraoperative PEX; afterwards 1.0–1.5 EPV.
- Substitution: albumin, FFP; initial intraoperative PEX 2 EPV albumin, 1 EPV FFP.
- Interval between procedures: approx. 48 h; after initial PEX, 5 PEX procedures are performed over 14 days.
- End of treatment: after final PEX, immunosuppression with IVIG 1 g/kg followed by ATG is performed.

Lung Transplant Rejection Graft rejection is a major factor for limiting lung transplant recipient survival. Rejection is classified as acute cell rejection (ACR), acute AbMR, and chronic rejection. Acute rejection presents with deteriorated pulmonary function tests, dyspnea, cough, and fatigue. Diagnosis also requires histologic evaluation, testing for DSA-HLA. Chronic rejection is a leading cause of death in lung transplant recipients. It may present with obstruction (e.g., bronchiolitis obliterans syndrome) or restrictive functional pattern (restrictive allograft syndrome) [17].

Treatment for acute cellular rejection includes high-dose steroids and ATG; acute AbMR is treated with steroids, Rituximab, IVIG, and PEX. Bronchiolitis obliterans syndrome is usually treated with high-dose steroids; ECP as well as ATG and alemtuzumab are used as second-line treatment [17].

The following ECP scheme is suggested in bronchiolitis obliterans syndrome [4]:

- Treatment volume per procedure (whole blood): 1.5 L (in-line ECP); 3–10 l (off-line ECP).
- Substitution: none.
- Frequency of treatment cycles: 12 treatment cycles in 6 months, initially 1 cycle per week.
- End of treatment: individualized, based on clinical improvement.

PEX treatment in acute AbMR in lung transplant [4]:

- Treatment volume: 1.0–1.5 EPV.
- Substitution: albumin, FFP.
- Interval between procedures: 24–48 h.
- End of treatment: clinical improvement.

References

1. Sorella A, Galanti K, Iezzi L, Gallina S, Mohammed SF, Sekhri N, et al. Diagnosis and management of dilated cardiomyopathy: a systematic review of clinical practice guidelines and recommendations. Eur Hear J Qual Care Clin Outcomes. 2025;11:206–22. https://doi.org/10.1093/ehjqcco/qcae109.
2. Hazebroek M, Dennert R, Heymans S. Idiopathic dilated cardiomyopathy: possible triggers and treatment strategies. Neth Hear J. 2012;20(7–8):332–5. https://doi.org/10.1007/s12471-012-0285-7.
3. Yoshikawa T, Baba A, Akaishi M, Wakabayashi Y, Monkawa T, Kitakaze M, et al. Immunoadsorption therapy for dilated cardiomyopathy using tryptophan column—a prospective, multicenter, randomized, within-patient and parallel-group comparative study to evaluate efficacy and safety. J Clin Apher. 2016;31(6):535–44. https://doi.org/10.1002/jca.21446.
4. Connelly-Smith L, Alquist CR, Aqui NA, Hofmann JC, Klingel R, Onwuemene OA, et al. Guidelines on the use of therapeutic apheresis in clinical practice—evidence-based approach from the writing Committee of the American Society for apheresis: the ninth special issue. J Clin Apher. 2023;38(2):77–278. https://doi.org/10.1002/jca.22043.

5. Peled Y, Ducharme A, Kittleson M, Bansal N, Stehlik J, Amdani S, et al. International Society for Heart and Lung Transplantation guidelines for the evaluation and care of cardiac transplant candidates—2024. J Hear Lung Transplant. 2024;43:1529–1628.e54. https://doi.org/10.1016/j.healun.2024.05.010.
6. Velleca A, Shullo MA, Dhital K, Azeka E, Colvin M, DePasquale E, et al. The International Society for Heart and Lung Transplantation (ISHLT) guidelines for the care of heart transplant recipients. J Heart Lung Transplant. 2023;42(5):e1–e141. https://doi.org/10.1016/j.healun.2022.10.015.
7. Pisani BA, Mullen GM, Malinowska K, Lawless CE, Mendez J, Silver MA, et al. Plasmapheresis with intravenous immunoglobulin G is effective in patients with elevated panel reactive antibody prior to cardiac transplantation. J Heart Lung Transplant. 1999;18(7):701–6. https://doi.org/10.1016/s1053-2498(99)00022-4.
8. Hurskainen M, Ainasoja O, Lemström KB. Failing heart transplants and rejection—a cellular perspective. J Cardiovasc Dev Dis. 2021;8(12):180. https://doi.org/10.3390/jcdd8120180.
9. Bruneval P, Angelini A, Miller D, Potena L, Loupy A, Zeevi A, et al. The XIIIth Banff conference on allograft pathology: the Banff 2015 heart meeting report: improving antibody-mediated rejection diagnostics: strengths, unmet needs, and future directions. Am J Transplant. 2017;17(1):42–53. https://doi.org/10.1111/ajt.14112.
10. Shu J, Santulli G. Update on peripheral artery disease: epidemiology and evidence-based facts. Atherosclerosis. 2018;275:379–81. https://doi.org/10.1016/j.atherosclerosis.2018.05.033.
11. Mazzolai L, Teixido-Tura G, Lanzi S, Boc V, Bossone E, Brodmann M, et al. ESC guidelines for the management of peripheral arterial and aortic diseases: developed by the task force on the management of peripheral arterial and aortic diseases of the European Society of Cardiology (ESC) endorsed by the European Association for Cardio-Thoracic Surgery (EACTS), the European reference network on rare multisystemic vascular diseases (VASCERN), and the European Society of Vascular Medicine (ESVM). Eur Heart J. 2024;45:3538–700. https://doi.org/10.1093/eurheartj/ehae179.
12. Berent T, Derfler K, Berent R, Sinzinger H. Lipoprotein apheresis in Austria—reduction of cardiovascular events by regular lipoprotein apheresis treatment. Atheroscler Suppl. 2019;40:8–11. https://doi.org/10.1016/j.atherosclerosissup.2019.08.025.
13. Ueda E, Ishiga K, Wakui H, Kawai Y, Kobayashi R, Kinguchi S, et al. Lipoprotein apheresis alleviates treatment-resistant peripheral artery disease despite the normal range of atherogenic lipoproteins: the LETS-PAD study. J Atheroscler Thromb. 2024;31:1370–85. https://doi.org/10.5551/jat.64639.

14. Adegunsoye A, Strek ME, Garrity E, Guzy R, Bag R. Comprehensive care of the lung transplant patient. Chest. 2017;152(1):150–64. https://doi.org/10.1016/j.chest.2016.10.001.
15. Aversa M, Martinu T, Patriquin C, Cypel M, Barth D, Ghany R, et al. Long-term outcomes of sensitized lung transplant recipients after peri-operative desensitization. Am J Transplant. 2021;21(10):3444–8. https://doi.org/10.1111/ajt.16707.
16. Tinckam KJ, Keshavjee S, Chaparro C, Barth D, Azad S, Binnie M, et al. Survival in sensitized lung transplant recipients with perioperative desensitization. Am J Transplant. 2015;15:417–26. https://doi.org/10.1111/ajt.13076.
17. Parulekar AD, Kao CC. Detection, classification, and management of rejection after lung transplantation. J Thorac Dis. 2019;11(Suppl 14):S1732–9. https://doi.org/10.21037/jtd.2019.03.83.

Plasma Exchange in Clinical Practice: Gastroenterology

9

Abstract

Plasma exchange (PEX) can be used as liver support system in acute liver failure (ALF), as well as desensitization protocols in liver transplantation. Other apheresis modalities are also used in gastroenterology, e.g., adsorptive cytapheresis (inflammatory bowel disease). Briefly the use of liver assist devices [molecular adsorbents recirculation system (MARS), fractionated plasma separation, and adsorption System (Prometheus) and single pass albumin dialysis (SPAD)] will be reviewed in ALF.

Keywords

Acute liver failure · Acute-on-chronic liver failure · Liver transplantation · Inflammatory bowel disease

Liver Failure: Acute and Acute-on-Chronic Liver Failure

Definition Acute liver failure (ALF) is a rare syndrome, associated with acute abnormality of liver blood tests in patients without preexisting chronic liver disease. The syndrome is characterized by hepatic coagulopathy and hepatic encephalopathy. Acute-on-

J. J. Filipov, *Therapeutic Plasma Exchange*, In Clinical Practice,
https://doi.org/10.1007/978-3-032-17275-4_9

chronic liver failure (ACLF) is a severe decompensation of preexisting liver disease, associated with high mortality and multiorgan failure (MOF) [1, 2].

Etiology and Pathophysiology ALF is caused by primary hepatocyte damage, due to viruses (hepatitis A, E, B), toxins, medications (Paracetamol, NSAIDs), and less frequently immune hepatitis, metabolic diseases (Wilson disease), and vascular disease (Budd-Chiari syndrome, hypoxic hepatitis). Massive liver damage causes liver failure; primary liver injury causes also inflammatory response, hemodynamic and metabolic abnormalities, causing multi-organ damage [1].

ACLF is a severe decompensated cirrhosis, characterized by multi-organ failure (brain, kidney, liver, coagulopathy, circulation, respiratory failure). MOF is triggered by infection, drug toxicity, and ischemia. Triggering factors cause systemic inflammation, leading to tissue hypoperfusion, immune-mediated tissue damage, and mitochondrial dysfunction [3].

Clinical Presentation

- ALF: liver damage (two- or threefold elevation of transaminases); impaired liver synthesis (jaundice and coagulopathy, INR > 1.5) and hepatic encephalopathy in cases without preexisting liver disease; yet acute presentation of autoimmune hepatitis and Budd-Chiari syndrome are exceptions to this rule. According to the time of development of hepatic encephalopathy from first sign of jaundice, ALF is categorized as hyperacute (within 7 days), acute (8–28 days), and subacute (5–12 weeks).
- ACLF: develops on top of acute decompensation of preexisting cirrhosis (e.g., acute development or worsening of ascites, encephalopathy, gastro-intestinal-hemorrhage, or combination of these), complicated with hepatic and extrahepatic organ failure [brain (hepatic encephalopathy), kidney (acute kidney injury), liver (jaundice), coagulation (INR ≥ 1.5), circulation (hypotension), respiration (respiratory failure)].

Treatment of ALF and ACLF

- ALF: supportive measures—cardiovascular (crystalloid infusions, vasopressors, hydrocortisone); respiratory (ventilation techniques); gastrointestinal support (nutrition, proton pump inhibitors); correction of biochemical abnormalities (e.g. hyponatremia); renal support—renal replacement therapy (RRT), continuous types preferred to intermittent RRT; treatment of infection; coagulation abnormalities correction (routine use of fresh frozen plasma is not recommended); neurological involvement—control of intracranial pressure, intubation, correction of metabolic abnormalities, earlier start of continuous RRT; liver failure—use of PEX and liver assist devices [artificial (e.g., Prometheus, MARS system) and bioartificial (using biological tissues—whole organ/hepatocyte cell lines). Artificial liver assist devices will be discussed later. It should be noted that charcoal hemoadsorption failed to improve patient survival in ALF. Finally, liver transplantation is a therapeutic option in ALF [1, 4].
- ACLF: treatment of precipitating factors (e.g., bacterial infection, hepatitis reactivation), nutritional support, organ support (e.g., RRT, ventilation techniques, vasopressors), liver transplantation. Liver assist devices, artificial or bioartificial, as well as PEX, are not recommended for routine use in ACLF, outside investigative trails [2].

Role of PEX and Liver Assist Devices in the Treatment of ALF and ACLF PEX as well as liver assist devices [single pass albumin dialysis (SPAD), Molecular Absorbent and Recirculating System (MARS®) and Fractionated Plasma Separation and Adsorption System (FPSA; Prometheus®, Fresenius, Germany)] were evaluated in the treatment of ALF and ACLF as bridging therapy to liver transplantation or hepatic recovery.

In ALF, PEX demonstrated better transplant-free survival, with improvement in ammonia and bilirubin levels and correction of coagulopathy. High-volume PEX (8–12 L PEX volume) is the reported PEX type. PEX treatment is more beneficial in patients, in which treatment is initiated early and who will not undergo liver transplantation [1, 4]. SPAD, MARS, and FPSA demonstrated improvement in ALF-associated hepatic encephalopathy but failed to improve mortality in ALF [5, 6]. None of these methods demonstrated superiority to the others [7]. Due to the conflicting results and insufficient evidence, current guidelines are not recommended for or against the routine use of high-volume PE or artificial liver support devices in ALF patients [4]. Charcoal adsorption also did not demonstrate survival benefit in ALF.

Current trials for ACLF demonstrate improvement in biochemical parameters, hepatic encephalopathy, and hemodynamic indicators from SPAD, MARS, FPSA; however, these methods do not achieve significant improvement in survival. PEX achieved improvement in 3-month survival; in the PROSPERO CRD42020155850 study, PEX demonstrated beneficial effect on mortality, in contrast to MARS and FPSA. The conflicting results, the heterogenous study groups, and low quality of evidence are limiting the routine use of PEX and liver assist devices in ACLF [7, 8].

PEX schedule in ALF/ACLF [4, 9]:

- Treatment volume per PEX: 1.0–1.5 EPV; in ALF, high-volume PEX (HVPEX, 8–12 L) is preferred.
- Substitution: FFP or FFP + albumin.
- Interval between sessions: 24 h.
- Target of treatment: clinical improvement or bridging to liver transplantation; most frequently three HVPEX sessions are performed,
- PEX is usually coupled with continuous renal replacement therapy (CRRT).

MARS treatment [10, 11]:

- Duration of MARS session: 6–8 h.
- Number of procedures: differs according to institution.
- Interval between sessions: usually 24 h or 48 h.
- Target of treatment: clinical improvement or bridging to liver transplantation.

SPAD treatment [7, 12]:

- Albumin dialysate: approx. 5000 ml; most frequently 4% albumin.
- Dialysate flow rate: 700–1000 ml/h; higher flow rate may have more beneficial result.
- Number of procedures: varies across institutions, similar to MARS.
- Interval between SPAD sessions: usually 24 h.
- Target of treatment: clinical improvement or bridging to liver transplantation.

FPSA treatment (Prometheus®, Fresenius, Germany) [13–16]:

- Duration of session: usually 6 h, minimum 4 h.
- Interval between sessions: varies, 24–48 h.
- Number of sessions: varies across institutions, ranging from 1 to 11 procedures.
- Target of treatment: clinical improvement or bridging to liver transplantation.

Liver Transplantation

Desensitization in Liver Transplantation (LT)

HLA sensitization and AB0 incompatibility are major obstacles to LT and are associated with poorer post-transplant survival [17, 18]. Desensitization protocols are particularly important in living donor LT; the benefit from their use in deceased donor LT is unclear.

ABO Incompatible (ABOi) Living Donor LT Desensitization in ABOi LT increases the donor pool and is of particular importance in living donation. PEX is used in combination with immunosuppressive treatment (e.g., Rituximab, RTX). Additionally, bortezomib may be added to the treatment if target iso-agglutinin titer is not achieved; IVIG can be added to the standard immunosuppression protocol. Apart from PEX, double filtration plasmapheresis (DFPP) was also used successfully in living donor AB0i LT [19].

PEX in AB0i LT [9, 20]:

- 2–3 weeks prior to LT—infuse Rituximab 375 mg/m^2.
- Start PEX 1 week prior LT.
- Treatment volume per PEX: 1–1.5 EPV.
- Substitution: albumin or FFP (donor and recipient compatible plasma).
- Interval between PEX: 24–48 h; usually 3 procedures within 7 days.
- Target of treatment: isoagglutinin titers ≤1:8; if target not achieved, additional immunosuppression with Bortezomib 1.3 mg/m^2 can be applied.

Donor Specific HLA Antibody (DSA-HLA) Desensitization in Living Donor LT Though hyperacute rejection due to preformed DSA-HLA antibodies is rare in LT, DSA-HLA are associated with poorer post-transplant outcomes.

Hong et al. demonstrated effective desensitization in living donor LT by applying Rituximab 375 mg/m^2 3 weeks, followed by 3 sessions of PEX 7 days prior to LT in patients with high antiglobulin T-cell cross match test (T-AHG) titers (≥1:16). Post-PEX T-AHG target titer was ˂1:16; if titers increased after LT above 1:64 in the post-transplant follow-up, additional PEX procedure was administered. Immunosuppressive therapy consisted of Basiliximab induction and triple maintenance immunosuppression (tacrolimus, mycophenolate, steroids) [21].

Additionally, PEX-free protocols were developed, targeting DSA-HLA desensitization, using RTX in cases with high mean fluorescence intensity (MFI >10,000) 2 weeks prior to LT; tacrolimus and mycophenolate were added to the immunosuppression 7 days prior to LT and IVIG post-transplant [22].

Suggested PEX schedule [9, 21]:

- 3 weeks prior to LT—infuse Rituximab 375 mg/m^2
- Start PEX 1 week prior LT.
- Treatment volume per PEX: 1–1.5 EPV.
- Substitution: albumin or FFP.
- Interval between PEX: 24–48 h; usually 3 procedures within 7 days.
- Target of treatment: ideally, negative cross-match; post-PEX T-AHG titer $<$1:16.

Liver Transplantation: Acute Rejection

Acute Antibody-Mediated Rejection (AbMR) in LT Generally, the incidence of acute AbMR after LT is lower, compared to other solid organ transplantations (e.g., heart and kidney). AbMR in LT resembles the treatment of acute AbMR in kidney transplantation [23].

Usually IVIG [100–500 mg/kg for 5 sessions (low dose), in some centers 2–5 g/kg (high dose)] and PEX are initiated; if the treatment is not effective, second-line treatment (e.g., RTX, Eculisumab) can be added. Maintenance immunosuppression should be optimized after treatment with PEX/IVIG [23].

Chronic AbMR in LT requires correction of maintenance immunosuppression or re-transplantation [24].

T-Cell Mediated Acute Rejection (TCMR) in LT Steroids are the first-line treatment in TCMR post-LT. However, if signs of accompanying AbMR are present, the abovementioned treatment options for AbMR can be used [24].

The following PEX schedule is suggested [9, 23, 24]:

- Immunosuppression is required: steroids, IVIG, RTX, bortezomib; maintenance immunosuppression optimization.
- Treatment volume per PEX: 1–1.5 EPV.
- Substitution: albumin or FFP.

- Interval between PEX: 24–48 h; usually 3 procedures within 7 days.
- Target of treatment: clinical and laboratory improvement.

Inflammatory Bowel Disease (IBD)

Definition IBD is a chronic inflammation of the guts, presenting with two subtypes: ulcerative colitis (UC), causing superficial mucosal inflammation that extends proximally and Crohn's disease (CD), associated with transmural inflammation of the bowel wall, and may affect any part of the gastro-intestinal system [25].

Pathogenesis and Pathophysiology Several risk factors have been established, linked to IBD. More than 200 genetic variants have been associated with affected recognition of microbial structures. Genetic predisposition is more pronounced in CD [25]. Microbial gut dysbiosis is also linked to IBD. Immune dysregulation (effector T-cells, regulatory T-cells, B-lymphocytes) is also implicated in pathophysiology of IBD. Finally, environmental factors (smoking, air pollution) may play a role in IBD pathogenesis [26].

Clinical Presentation

- CD: abdominal pain, diarrhea, and fatigue and weight loss, fever; CD is complicated with recurrent fistulas, anemia, and impaired growth. Extrarenal involvement may be present—arthropathy, ocular, hepatobiliary, and thrombotic manifestations. CD is diagnosed clinically, based on laboratory and instrumental findings [27].
- UC: rectal bleeding, increased bowel movement/stool frequency; it can be complicated with toxic megacolon. Similar extrarenal manifestations may be detected. Diagnosis requires also instrumental and laboratory tests [28].

Treatment of IBD. Role of Adsorptive Cytapheresis Currently, steroids (systemic or locally acting), methotrexate, thiopurines (e.g., azathiorpine), TNFα antagonists (e.g., infliximab, adalimumab), interleukin (IL) 12/23 inhibitors, anti-integrin molecules, and Janus kinase inhibitors are used for induction therapy and/or maintenance treatment in CD and UC [27–30].

Adsorptive cytapheresis (ACP) is a procedure, in which a special filter is used to adsorb certain cell populations. Technically, the blood is drawn from the patient; it flows into specialized filter, absorbing certain WBC (granulocytes, monocytes, lymphocytes) and platelets. Afterwards the blood is returned to the patient. After removal of inflammatory cells, inflammatory mediators are downregulated; thus, inflammatory process is being suppressed. With the introduction of novel treatment options in IBD, ACP has limited use, mainly in resistant cases.

The following treatment schedule in UC/CD is suggested [9, 31]:

- Treatment volume: blood volume varies (1800 or 3000 ml) according to type of ACP equipment.
- Interval between ACP sessions: 1 week; more intensive approach as induction therapy (2 sessions per week) may be used, followed by maintenance ACP 2 sessions monthly for up to 14 maintenance sessions.
- Target of treatment: clinical improvement; 5 to 10 sessions may be required for induction therapy; maintenance dose varies across different institutions.

References

1. European Association for the Study of the Liver. EASL clinical practical guidelines on the management of acute (fulminant) liver failure. J Hepatol. 2017;66(5):1047–81. https://doi.org/10.1016/j.jhep.2016.12.003.
2. Moreau R, Tonon M, Krag A, Angeli P, Berenguer M, Berzigotti A, et al. EASL clinical practice guidelines on acute-on-chronic liver failure. J Hepatol. 2023;79(2):461–91. https://doi.org/10.1016/j.jhep.2023.04.021.

3. Zaccherini G, Weiss E, Moreau R. Acute-on-chronic liver failure: definitions, pathophysiology and principles of treatment. JHEP Rep. 2021;3(1):100176. https://doi.org/10.1016/j.jhepr.2020.100176.
4. Shingina A, Mukhtar N, Wakim-Fleming J, Alqahtani S, Wong RJ, Limketkai BN, et al. Acute liver failure guidelines. Am J Gastroenterol. 2023;118:1128–53. https://doi.org/10.14309/ajg.0000000000002340.
5. Tsipotis E, Shuja A, Jaber BL. Albumin dialysis for liver failure: a systematic review. Adv Chronic Kidney Dis. 2015;22(5):382–90. https://doi.org/10.1053/j.ackd.2015.05.004.
6. Gadour E, Kaballo MA, Shrwani K, Hassan Z, Kotb A, Aljuraysan A, et al. Safety and efficacy of Single-Pass Albumin Dialysis (SPAD), Prometheus, and Molecular Adsorbent Recycling System (MARS) liver haemodialysis vs. Standard Medical Therapy (SMT): meta-analysis and systematic review. Prz Gastroenterol. 2024;19:101–11. https://doi.org/10.5114/pg.2024.139297.
7. García Martínez JJ, Bendjelid K. Artificial liver support systems: what is new over the last decade? Ann Intensive Care. 2018;8(1):109. https://doi.org/10.1186/s13613-018-0453-z.
8. Ocskay K, Kanjo A, Gede N, Szakács Z, Pár G, Erőss B, et al. Uncertainty in the impact of liver support systems in acute-on-chronic liver failure: a systematic review and network meta-analysis. Ann Intensive Care. 2021;11(1):10. https://doi.org/10.1186/s13613-020-00795-0.
9. Connelly-Smith L, Alquist CR, Aqui NA, Hofmann JC, Klingel R, Onwuemene OA, et al. Guidelines on the use of therapeutic apheresis in clinical practice—evidence-based approach from the writing Committee of the American Society for apheresis: the ninth special issue. J Clin Apher. 2023;38(2):77–278. https://doi.org/10.1002/jca.22043.
10. Gerth HU, Pohlen M, Thölking G, Pavenstädt H, Brand M, Wilms C, et al. Molecular adsorbent recirculating system (MARS) in acute liver injury and graft dysfunction: results from a case-control study. PLoS One. 2017;12(4):e0175529. https://doi.org/10.1371/journal.pone.0175529.
11. Boyle M, Kurtovic J, Bihari D, Riordan S, Steiner C. Equipment review: the molecular adsorbents recirculating system (MARS®). Crit Care. 2004;8(4):280–6. https://doi.org/10.1186/cc2895.
12. Sponholz C, Matthes K, Rupp D, Backaus W, Klammt S, Karailieva D, et al. Molecular adsorbent recirculating system and single-pass albumin dialysis in liver failure – a prospective, randomised crossover study. Crit Care. 2016;20:2. https://doi.org/10.1186/s13054-015-1159-3.
13. Kribben A, Gerken G, Haag S, Hergetrosenthal S, Treichel U, Betz C, et al. Effects of fractionated plasma separation and adsorption on survival in patients with acute-on-chronic liver failure. Gastroenterology. 2012;142(4):782–789.e3. https://doi.org/10.1053/j.gastro.2011.12.056.
14. Şentürk E, Esen F, Özcan PE, Rifai K, Pinarbaşi B, Çakar N, et al. The treatment of acute liver failure with fractionated plasma separation and

adsorption system: experience in 85 applications. J Clin Apher. 2010;25(4):195–201. https://doi.org/10.1002/jca.20238.

15. Komardina E, Yaroustovsky M, Abramyan M, Plyushch M. Prometheus therapy for the treatment of acute liver failure in patients after cardiac surgery. Pol J Cardiovasc Thorac Surg. 2017;14(4):230–5. https://doi.org/10.5114/kitp.2017.72226.
16. Rifai K, Ernst T, Kretschmer U, Bahr MJ, Schneider A, Hafer C, et al. Prometheus® – a new extracorporeal system for the treatment of liver failure. J Hepatol. 2003;39(6):984–90. https://doi.org/10.1016/s0168-8278(03)00468-9.
17. Goto R, Ito M, Kawamura N, Watanabe M, Ganchiku Y, Kamiyama T, et al. The impact of preformed donor-specific antibodies in living donor liver transplantation according to graft volume. Immunity Inflamm Dis. 2022;10(3):e586. https://doi.org/10.1002/iid3.586.
18. Gan K, Li Z, Bao S, Fang Y, Wang T, Jin L, et al. Clinical outcomes after ABO-incompatible liver transplantation: a systematic review and meta-analysis. Transpl Immunol. 2021;69:101476. https://doi.org/10.1016/j.trim.2021.1014761.
19. Bajpai M, Kakkar B, Gupta S, Rastogi A, Pamecha V. Cascade plasmapheresis as a desensitization strategy for patients undergoing ABO incompatible living donor liver transplantation (ABOi LDLT): a single center experience. Transfus Apher Sci. 2019;58(4):442–6. https://doi.org/10.1016/j.transci.2019.04.028.
20. Lee TB, Ko HJ, Shim JR, Choi BH, Ryu JH, Yang K. Abo-incompatible living donor liver transplantation with a simplified desensitization and immunosuppression protocol: a single-center retrospective study. Exp Clin Transplant. 2021;19(7):676–85. https://doi.org/10.6002/ect.2021.0025.
21. Hong G, Yi NJ, Suh S, Won YT, Kim H, Park MS, et al. Preoperative selective desensitization of live donor liver transplant recipients considering the degree of T lymphocyte cross-match titer, model for end-stage liver disease score, and graft liver volume. J Korean Med Sci. 2014;29(5):640–7.
22. Ogawa K, Tamura K, Sakamoto K, Funamizu N, Honjo M, Shine M, et al. Living donor liver transplantation in patients with preformed donor-specific anti-human leukocyte antigen antibodies using preoperative desensitization therapy according to intensity of donor-specific antibodies: a single-center study. Ann Transplant. 2023;28:e941346. https://doi.org/10.12659/AOT.941346.
23. Lee BT, Fiel MI, Schiano TD. Antibody-mediated rejection of the liver allograft: an update and a clinico-pathological perspective. J Hepatol. 2021;75(5):1203–16. https://doi.org/10.1016/j.jhep.2021.07.027.
24. De Martin E, Berg T, Berenguer M, Burra P, Fondevila C, Heimbach JK, et al. EASL clinical practice guidelines on liver transplantation. J Hepatol [Internet]. 2024;81:1040–86. https://doi.org/10.1016/j.jhep.2024.07.032.

25. Chang JT. Pathophysiology of inflammatory bowel disease. N Engl J Med. 2020;383:2652–64. https://doi.org/10.1056/NEJMra2002697.
26. Zhang YZ, Li YY. Inflammatory bowel disease: pathogenesis. World J Gastroenterol. 2014;20(1):91–9. https://doi.org/10.3748/wjg.v20.i1.91.
27. Lichtenstein GR, Loftus EV, Afzali A, Long MD, Barnes EL, Isaacs KL, et al. ACG clinical guideline: management of Crohn's disease in adults. Am J Gastroenterol. 2025;120(6):1225–64. https://doi.org/10.14309/ajg.0000000000003465.
28. Rubin DT, Ananthakrishnan AN, Siegel CA, Barnes ELM, Long MD. ACG clinical guideline: ulcerative colitis in adults. Am J Gastroenterol. 2025;120(6):1187–224. https://doi.org/10.14309/ajg.0000000000003463.
29. Gordon H, Minozzi S, Kopylov U, Verstockt B, Chaparro M, Buskens C, et al. ECCO guidelines on therapeutics in Crohn's disease: medical treatment. J Crohns Colitis. 2024;18:1531–55. https://doi.org/10.1093/ecco-jcc/jjae091.
30. Raine T, Bonovas S, Burisch J, Kucharzik T, Adamina M, Annese V, et al. ECCO guidelines on therapeutics in ulcerative colitis: medical treatment. J Crohns Colitis. 2022;16(1):2–17. https://doi.org/10.1093/ecco-jcc/jjab178.
31. Ueno N, Kobayashi Y, Sakatani A, Dokoshi T, Takahashi K, Ando K, et al. Granulocyte and monocyte adsorptive apheresis maintenance therapy restored the loss of response to anti-TNF-alpha agents in the patients with UC: a case report. J Clin Apher. 2025;40:1–5. https://doi.org/10.1002/jca.70030.

Plasma Exchange in Clinical Practice: Oncology and Sepsis

10

Abstract

Plasma exchange is usually implied in the treatment of neoplasia complications (e.g., malignancy-associated thrombotic microangiopathy, paraneoplastic syndromes, hyperviscosity syndrome) and drug-associated adverse events (e.g., cisplatin toxicity, drug-induced thrombotic microangiopathy). Apheresis modalities are rarely used for the treatment of malignancy itself (e.g., extracorporeal photopheresis in Sézary syndrome). Plasma exchange and hemoadsorption are not routinely recommended in the treatment of sepsis due to conflicting results from trials and low quality of evidence.

Keywords

Paraneoplastic syndromes · Hyperviscosity syndrome · Mycosis fungoides · Cisplatin · Immune check-point inhibitors · Sepsis

Plasma Exchange in the Treatment of Solid Tumors

Complications from solid tumors are generally indications for PEX in solid neoplasms.

J. J. Filipov, *Therapeutic Plasma Exchange*, In Clinical Practice,
https://doi.org/10.1007/978-3-032-17275-4_10

Paraneoplastic Syndromes (PNPS)

Definition Paraneoplastic syndromes are rare systemic manifestations of malignancy, due to production of antibodies, hormones, and peptides by the tumor. Multiple systems can be involved, presenting with endocrine, neurological, skin, cardiovascular symptoms. The etiology of paraneoplastic syndromes is associated with cancers (e.g., small cell lung cancer, breast cancer, gynecological cancers, thymomas) [1].

Clinical Presentation

- Endocrine syndromes: hypercalcemia, Cushing syndrome, syndrome of inappropriate anti-diuretidin hormone secretion (SIADH), hypoglycemia.
- Neurological syndromes: limbic encephalitis, cerebellar degeneration, myasthenia gravis, autonomic neuropathy, subacute sensorial neuropathy.
- Skin manifestations: dermatomyositis, acanthosis nigricans, paraneoplastic pemphigus, leukocytoclastic vasculitis, Trousseau syndrome.
- Rheumatologic syndromes: paraneoplastic polyarthritis, polymyalgia rheumatic, hypertrophic osteoarthropathy.
- Ocular symptoms: cancer-associated retinopathy, cancer-associated cone dysfunction.
- Renal symptoms: nephritic syndrome, electrolyte abnormalities.
- Hematological symptoms: polycythemia.

Treatment of PNPS. Role of PEX The major goal in controlling PNPS is the therapy of the primary disease. Unfortunately, PNPS may present earlier than the tumor itself, requiring broad differential diagnosis in this case and earlier neoplasia detection. Treatment of primary tumor is associated with improvement in PNPS.

Usually symptomatic treatments, e.g., correction of electrolyte disorders, correction of edema, hypoglycemia treatment, and hormonal therapy, are required for endocrine manifestations.

Particularly important are immune-mediated PNPS—neurological, ocular, and skin, due to antibody-mediated cross-reaction against tumor antigens and normal molecules in the central nervous system, skin, and eyes. In these cases, immunosuppression (high-dose steroids, azathioprine, Rituximab, cyclophosphamide, IVIG) can be applied [1].

PEX can be added to the immunosuppressive treatment; however, it is not a first-line treatment in PNPS and may be used in refractory cases. Unfortunately, PEX, combined with immunosuppression or chemotherapy, failed to demonstrate long-lasting effect on antibody titers and failed to achieve stable clinical resolution of PNPS [2]. Additionally, immunoadsorption may be used in PNPS [3].

- PEX volume: 1–1.5 EPV.
- Substitution: albumin.
- Interval between PEX: 24–48 h.
- Treatment target: clinical improvement.

Malignancy-Associated Thrombotic Microangiopathy (mTMA)

Definition Malignancy-associated TMA (mTMA) ranges clinically from asymptomatic laboratory findings to overt complement-mediated TMA or thrombotic thrombocytopenic purpura (TTP) and usually is due to neoplasia itself or a complication of antineoplastic therapy/superimposed infection [4].

Pathogenesis Malignancy causes mTMA itself, typically in mucin-secreting and metastatic malignancies (most commonly gastro-intestinal, breast, prostate, and lung cancers). Tumor cells can directly activate clotting factors; tumor bone marrow invasion can also cause endothelial injury, which in turn leads to production of vWF multimers. ADAMTS 13 activity may be decreased too, but it is usually normal or mildly reduced in mTMA [4, 5]. Secondly, mTMA can be caused by chemotherapy and immune therapies.

Clinical Presentation mTMA should be distinguished from other TMAs and other malignancy-associated complications. Patients tend to be older, and pulmonary symptoms are more frequent in mTMA; signs for active malignancy should be sought. In addition, mTMA is frequently associated with metastatic cancers. ADAMTS 13 activity is not severely reduced unlike primary TTP. Symptoms usually have longer duration in mTMA [5].

Treatment. Role of PEX Currently no consensus on the treatment exists. Generally, if mTMA is caused by medication, the drug should be stopped. Immunosuppressive treatment has no clear benefit.

Primary goal and most effective approach in mTMA resolution remains treatment of primary neoplasia (surgical/chemotherapy) [6].

PEX failed to demonstrate clear benefit in mTMA [4]. However, it may be useful in TTP and low ADAMTS 13 activity; therefore, PEX may be initiated until ADAMTS 13 results are present; malignancy diagnosis should be performed too, as primary disease treatment can effectively prolong patient's life [6, 7].

As previously mentioned, no current consensus on PEX use in mTMA exists and no clear benefit from PEX in mTMA has been established. Timely diagnosis and treatment of cancer play a pivotal role. However, based on the recommendations for other types of TMA, the following PEX schedule can be considered:

- Treatment volume per PEX: 1.0–1.5 EPV.
- Interval between PEX procedures: 24 h.
- Substitution: fresh frozen plasma (FFP) + albumin, FFP only in low ADAMTS 13 activity.
- Target of treatment: clinical and laboratory improvement; malignancy diagnosis and primary disease treatment should be prioritized.

Plasma Exchange in the Treatment of Hematological Tumors

Hyperviscosity Syndrome

Definition Hyperviscosity syndrome (HVS) is a rare complication of hematological malignancy, associated with increased blood viscosity due to increased immunoglobulin synthesis (monoclonal/polyclonal), e.g., multiple myeloma and Waldenström's disease, or increased blood cell count [red blood cells (RBC), white blood cells (WBC), less frequently platelets(PLT)], most frequently due to acute leukemia or polycythemia vera.

Clinical Manifestation HVS has several major syndromes [8]:

- Neurological disturbances: seizures, coma or somnolence, cerebral hemorrhage.
- Ocular symptoms: blurred vision, papilledema, bilateral retinal hemorrhage/thrombosis.
- Mucosal bleeding.
- Cardiac symptoms: high output heart failure.

Treatment of HVS. Role of PEX Treatment of HVS includes treatment of primary disease (chemotherapy) and symptomatic treatment (e.g., hydration in myeloma nephropathy). Additionally, different apheresis techniques can be applied:

- PEX—in myeloma nephropathy, hypergammaglobulinemia (Waldenström's disease).
- Leukocytapheresis—acute leukemia.
- Erythrocytapheresis—polycytemia vera.
- Thrombocytapheresis—primary thrombocytosis.

Their use and effectiveness are discussed in detail in Chap. 4.

Mycosis Fungoides and Sézary Syndrome

Definition Mycosis fungoides (MF) is a form of cutaneous T-cell lymphoma, characterized by epidermotropism of clonal T-cells. Its erythrodermic form presents with generalized erythema. The systemic subtype of cutaneous T-cell lymphoma is referred as Sézary syndrome (SS), characterized by detecting pathological Sézary cells in peripheral blood.

Clinical Presentation MF presents with skin involvement (dermatitis-like patches, erythema) and has a chronic course. In SS, skin involvement is present (erythema, affecting more than 80% of body surface) along with lymph node involvement and high burden of pathognomonic Sézary cells ≥1000/μl [9].

Treatment of MF and SS Two major aspects of MF and SS treatment exist—local, skin-oriented therapy (topical steroids, chlormetine, UV therapy, photodynamic therapy) and systemic treatment, usually used in resistant local therapy and advanced stages of MF and SS (retinoids, IFNα, chemotherapy, targeted immunotherapy, as well as extracorporeal photopheresis, ECP).

ECP is regarded as first-line treatment in advanced erythrodermic MF or SS, either alone or in combination with other therapies (local and systemic). Extracorporeal photopheresis is based on centrifugal leukocytapheresis. After separating the WBC by centrifugation, they are treated with 8-methoxypsoralen, which is added to the effluent. Separated WBC, treated with 8-methoxypsoralen are exposed to ultraviolet A light and are returned to the patient. Two types of ECP are present—in-line ECP, in which UVA radiation occurs during the centrifugation of leukocytes, and off-line ECP, in which WBC separation and UV radiation occur in different devices, so the patient is disconnected from the separation device once WBC separation is accomplished. In-line ECP processes 1.5 L of blood, 2 procedures in 2 consecutive days are regarded as one cycle; in off-line, ECP larger volumes are processed (3.5–10 L).

ECP treatment schedule in MF/SS [3, 10]:

- Interval between treatment cycles: 2–4 weeks, higher frequency may be used in the first 3 months.
- Treatment duration: 5–10 months.
- Treatment target: clinical improvement; maintenance treatment can be applied.

PEX in the Treatment of Anti-neoplastic Drug Toxicity

Cisplatin Overdose

Cisplatin is a heavy metal-based antitumor drug that binds to serum proteins. Cisplatin toxicity comprises of bone marrow suppression, vomiting, organ toxicity, including hearing loss; due to the high percentage of serum protein binding, the drug may have longer duration of toxicity and is not effectively removed by hemodialysis [11]. Several reports have demonstrated effective reduction in cisplatin levels and effective resolution of overdose symptoms after PEX, either alone or in combination of other therapeutic methods (dialysis and supportive treatment); however, clearly defined guideline on the use of PEX in cisplatin toxicity does not exist. The following PEX schedule is suggested [12, 13]:

- Treatment volume per PEX: 1.0–1.5 EPV.
- Interval between PEX procedures: 24–48 h.
- Substitution: albumin, FFP.
- Target of treatment: clinical and laboratory improvement.

Antineoplastic Drug-Induced TMA (diTMA)

Several antineoplastic agents can cause diTMA: Gemcitabine, Mitomycin, Sunitinib, Vincristine [14]. Generally, two major mechanisms for diTMA exist—direct toxicity and immune-mediated injury, causing endothelial damage, overactivation of the complement system, suppression of ADAMTS 13 activity, and finally microthrombi formation. Treatment cessation, accompanied by immunosuppression, is the initial step in antineoplastic diTMA. PEX has unclear benefit in antineoplastic diTMA; in Gemcitabine-associated TMA, its use is not recommended.

Suggested therapeutic schedule [3]:

- Treatment volume per PEX: 1.0–1.5 EPV.
- Interval between PEX procedures: 24 h.
- Substitution: FFP or FFP + albumin.
- Target treatment: PEX to continue until normal PLT count for at least 2 consecutive days has been achieved.

Immune-Related Adverse Effects from Immune Check-Point Inhibitors (ICI)

ICI are a novel group of antitumor monoclonal antibody therapy, targeting checkpoint molecules [programmed death-1 (PD-1), programmed death-ligand 1 (PD-L1), and cytotoxic T-lymphocyte-associated protein 4 (CTLA-4)], thus boosting antitumor reaction to cancer. ICI have improved significantly outcomes in several cancers and melanoma [15]. Their effectiveness has been limited due to ICI resistance and immune-related adverse events.

Immune-related adverse events include a wide range of symptoms and involve different organs: central nervous system (myasthenia gravis), endocrine (diabetes. thyroiditis); cardiac (myocarditis), musculoskeletal (myositis), and hematological (thrombotic thrombocytopenic purpira (TTP)). The first-line treatment is drug cessation and immunosuppression (steroids, RTX, and tacrolimus) [16].

In resistant cases PEX can be considered. The following therapeutic scheme is suggested [3]:

- Treatment volume per PEX: 1.0–1.5 EPV.
- Interval between PEX procedures: 24–48 h.
- Substitution: albumin, FFP. Albumin substitution is preferred.
- Target of treatment: clinical and laboratory improvement.

- In cases of ICI-associated TTP and myasthenia gravis, the respective therapeutic schedules should be applied (see Chaps. 4 and 6).

Plasma Exchange in the Treatment of Sepsis

Definition Sepsis is defined as life-threatening organ dysfunction, due to abnormal host response to infection [17]. Despite improvement in outcomes over the last decades, it remains a major cause for death worldwide.

Clinical Manifestation Currently a specific assessment tools have been created to evaluate the presence of sepsis, namely, sepsis-related organ failure assessment (SOFA) tool, incorporating respiratory, cardiovascular abnormalities (partial oxygen pressure, mean arterial pressure need for vasopressors), coagulation pathology (low platelet count) CNS changes (Glasgow coma score change), abnormal liver, and kidney tests (including decreased urine output) [17].

Treatment of Sepsis. Role of PEX Currently the major aspects in sepsis treatment are antibiotics, fluid resuscitation, vasopressor agents if low mean arterial pressure is present despite fluid resuscitation, albumin infusion, renal replacement treatment, venoarterial extracorporeal membrane oxygenation (VA-ECMO) in cases with septic shock, who fail to respond to other treatment options [18].

PEX and other apheresis modalities (hemoadsorption) have been evaluated in the treatment of sepsis, but the results from the studies are conflicting (especially in terms of mortality reduction) and the level of evidence in some of the published trials is low [19]. The following therapeutic schedule is suggested [3]:

- Treatment volume per PEX: 1.0–1.5 EPV.
- Interval between PEX procedures: 24 h.
- Substitution: FFP.
- Target of treatment: clinical and laboratory improvement.

However, due to the conflicting results PEX is not part of the routine sepsis treatment [18]. Recent guidelines also suggested against the use of polymyxin B hemoadsorption in sepsis; the routine use of other apheresis techniques in sepsis was not recommended due to insufficient evidence too [20].

References

1. Pelosof LC, Gerber DE. Paraneoplastic syndromes: an approach to diagnosis and treatment. Mayo Clin Proc. 2010;85(9):838–54. https://doi.org/10.4065/mcp.2010.0099.
2. Chiu D, Rhee J, Gonzalez Castro LN. Diagnosis and treatment of paraneoplastic neurologic syndromes. Antibodies (Basel). 2023;12(3):50. https://doi.org/10.3390/antib12030050.
3. Connelly-Smith L, Alquist CR, Aqui NA, Hofmann JC, Klingel R, Onwuemene OA, et al. Guidelines on the use of therapeutic apheresis in clinical practice—evidence-based approach from the writing committee of the American Society for Apheresis: the ninth special issue. J Clin Apher. 2023;38(2):77–278. https://doi.org/10.1002/jca.22043.
4. Font C, de Herreros MG, Tsoukalas N, Brito-Dellan N, Espósito F, Escalante C, et al. Thrombotic microangiopathy (TMA) in adult patients with solid tumors: a challenging complication in the era of emerging anticancer therapies. Support Care Cancer. 2022;30(10):8599–609. https://doi.org/10.1007/s00520-022-06935-5.
5. Babu KG, Bhat GR. Cancer-associated thrombotic microangiopathy. Ecancermedicalscience. 2016;10:1–11. https://doi.org/10.3332/ecancer.2016.649.
6. Winters JL. Plasma exchange in thrombotic microangiopathies (TMAs) other than thrombotic thrombocytopenic purpura (TTP). Hematology. 2017;2017(1):632–8. https://doi.org/10.1182/asheducation-2017.1.632.
7. Lechner K, Obermeier HL. Cancer-related microangiopathic hemolytic anemia: clinical and laboratory features in 168 reported cases. Medicine (Baltimore). 2012;91(4):195–205. https://doi.org/10.1097/MD.0b013e3182603598.
8. Gertz MA. Acute hyperviscosity: syndromes and management. Blood. 2018;132(13):1379–85. https://doi.org/10.1182/blood-2018-06-846816.
9. Latzka J, Assaf C, Bagot M, Cozzio A, Dummer R, Guenova E, et al. EORTC consensus recommendations for the treatment of mycosis fungoides/Sézary syndrome—Update 2023. Eur J Cancer. 2023;195:113343. https://doi.org/10.1016/j.ejca.2023.113343.
10. Knobler R, Arenberger P, Arun A, Assaf C, Bagot M, Berlin G, et al. European dermatology forum—updated guidelines on the use of extra-

corporeal photopheresis 2020—part 1. J. Eur. Acad. Dermatology Venereol. 2020;34(12):2693–716. https://doi.org/10.1111/jdv.16890.

11. Hu Y, Yang H, Fu S, Wu J. Therapeutic plasma exchange: for cancer patients. Cancer Manag Res. 2022;14:411–25. https://doi.org/10.2147/CMAR.S340472.
12. Jung HK, Lee J, Lee SN. A case of massive cisplatin overdose managed by plasmapheresis. Korean J Intern Med. 1995;10(2):150–4. https://doi.org/10.3904/kjim.1995.10.2.150.
13. Hofmann G, Bauernhofer T, Krippl P, Lang-Loidolt D, Horn S, Goessler W, et al. Plasmapheresis reverses all side-effects of a cisplatin overdose – a case report and treatment recommendation. BMC Cancer. 2006;6:1. https://doi.org/10.1186/1471-2407-6-1.
14. Al-Nouri ZL, Reese JA, Terrell DR, Vesely SK, George JN. Drug-induced thrombotic microangiopathy: a systematic review of published reports. Blood. 2015;125:616–8. https://doi.org/10.1182/blood-2014-11-611335.
15. Meng L, Wu H, Wu J, Ding P, He J, Sang M, et al. Mechanisms of immune checkpoint inhibitors: insights into the regulation of circular RNAS involved in cancer hallmarks. Cell Death Dis. 2024;15(1):3. https://doi.org/10.1038/s41419-023-06389-5.
16. Haanen J, Obeid M, Spain L, Carbonnel F, Wang Y, Robert C, et al. Management of toxicities from immunotherapy: ESMO clinical practice guideline for diagnosis, treatment and follow-up. Ann Oncol. 2022;33(12):1217–38. https://doi.org/10.1016/j.annonc.2022.10.001.
17. Singer M, Deutschman CS, Seymour C, Shankar-Hari M, Annane D, Bauer M, et al. The third international consensus definitions for sepsis and septic shock (sepsis-3). JAMA – J. Am. Med. Assoc. 2016;315(8):801–10. https://doi.org/10.1001/jama.2016.0287.
18. Carvey MM, Glauser J. The management of severe sepsis and septic shock: a novel update and bedside reference guide. Curr Emerg Hosp Med Rep. 2025;13(7) https://doi.org/10.1007/s40138-025-00310-4.
19. Pisano A, Venditto M, Palmieri C, Landoni G. Novel therapies and interventions in sepsis and septic shock. BJA Educ. 2025;25:206–17. https://doi.org/10.1016/j.bjae.2025.01.003.
20. Evans L, Rhodes A, Alhazzani W, Antonelli M, Coopersmith CM, French C, et al. Surviving sepsis campaign: international guidelines for management of sepsis and septic shock 2021. Intensive Care Med. 2021;47(11):1181–247. https://doi.org/10.1007/s00134-021-06506-y.

Drug Removal in PEX

11

Abstract

Drug removal by PEX depends on pharmacokinetics of each drug, as well as on PEX characteristics (duration, frequency, volume) and clinical parameters for each patient (malnutrition, organ dysfunction). The data on drug removal by plasma exchange and other apheresis techniques are limited, and published studies have low quality of evidence due to small number of patients (often case reports), heterogeneity (different clinical scenarios, treatment of poisoning vs evaluation of drug removal), different apheresis techniques, and different pharmacokinetics of the evaluated agents. The chapter evaluates different factors for drug removal and gives guide on medication use in PEX.

Keywords

Volume of distribution (Vd) · Protein binding affinity · Drug clearance

J. J. Filipov, *Therapeutic Plasma Exchange*, In Clinical Practice,
https://doi.org/10.1007/978-3-032-17275-4_11

General Principles of Medication Removal in PEX

During plasma exchange, patient's plasma is separated from blood cellular elements and is substituted by human albumin and/or FFP. Thus, protein-bound medications can be removed from the body by PEX, and their effectiveness may be significantly changed due to direct drug removal or due to medication—metabolizing enzyme removal [1]. Though the main factors for drug removal in PEX evaluated in literature are protein binding (>80%) and low volume of distribution (Vd) of the medication (Vd˂0.2 L/kg), several other important determinants of PEX-associated drug removal exist. Generally, these factors are medication-associated and clinical/technical ones [2]. As PEX-associated removal is not influenced by a single parameter, exact prediction about the extent of drug removal is often difficult to evaluate.

Medication-Associated Factors

Generally, larger intravascular distribution is required for significant PEX-associated drug removal. The following pharmacokinetic parameters are considered:

- Volume of distribution (*Vd*): represents the tendency of a drug to remain in the plasma or distribute in other tissues. *Vd* is expressed via the following equation:

$$Vd\left(L\right)=\frac{\text{Amount of drug in the body}\left(\text{mg}\right)}{\text{Plasma drug concentration}\left(\text{mg / L}\right)} \tag{11.1}$$

Vd can be expressed in L/kg, when normalized to body weight. Larger *Vd* corresponds to greater tissue distribution, whereas lower *Vd* corresponds to higher plasma distribution. *Vd*˂0.2 L/kg indicates high intravascular distribution and high probability for PEX removal [2].

- Protein binding affinity: higher protein binding (>80%) is associated with higher intravascular distribution and therefore higher risk for PEX removal.
- Half-life ($T_{1/2}$) (see Eq. 11.2) and endogenous clearance: longer $T_{1/2}$ and lower endogenous clearance indicate longer elimination of the medication, thus providing higher plasma concentrations for a longer period of time. $T_{1/2}$ longer than 2 h and endogenous clearance lower than 4 ml/min (0.24 L/hour).

$$Half-life(hour) = 0.693 * \frac{Vd(L)}{Clearance(L/hour)} \quad (11.2)$$

- Time interval between drug application and initiation of PEX: Associated with the multi-compartment drug distribution, there are two phases in medication metabolism: distribution phase, in which the medication leaves the plasma and is distributed to peripheral tissues; and elimination phase, in which the drug returns to the plasma and is eliminated from the body [3]. In medications with multi-compartment distribution model, a PEX procedure within the distribution phase is associated with increased risk for its removal. Medications, applied prior to PEX, may achieve maximal concentration prior to the procedure, and as redistribution to other tissues occurs, their removal by PEX will be insignificant if the time interval is long enough between their application and PEX. Therefore, an adequate PEX timing after the distribution phase is required. For example, Cefepime has low *Vd* (approx. 0.2 L/kg), low protein binding (20%) and $T_{1/2}$ of 2 h and achieves maximal concentration 30 min after intravenous application. Yet a study demonstrated insignificant PEX removal of the antibiotic if the procedure was initiated 2 h after intravenous application of 2 grams Cefepime [4, 5].
- Hydrophilic/lipophilic active molecule.

Clinical and Technical Factors

Clinical Factors, Influencing Drug Removal in PEX The following clinical situations may influence medication removal in PEX [2]:

- Nutritional status.
- Organ damage, affecting drug metabolism (e.g., liver or kidney disease).
- Patient instability: e.g., hypotension lowers PEX-associated removal (valid for intoxications).

Technical Factors [2, 6] Type of apheresis [PEX, lipoprotein apheresis, hemoadsorption, red blood cells (RBC) exchange].

- Procedure duration.
- Frequency of PEX.
- Type of substitution fluid: its importance is mainly in the cases of toxic drug levels. Generally, albumin solutions are preferred for drug removal. However, certain medications bind specifically to specific plasma proteins, requiring the use of FFP. For example, quinidine, propranolol, and chlorpromazine bind to alpha-1-acid glycoprotein, thus making FFP the preferred option for substitution in these types of intoxications.

Drug Clearance in Other Apheresis Techniques

Due to the different structure (hydrophilic vs lipophilic) and different tissue distribution, medications may be removed by other apheresis modalities, e.g., lipoprotein apheresis. However, the data for drug removal in other apheresis types is scarce, as most of the papers demonstrate results in plasma exchange.

Lipoprotein Apheresis(LA) In LA lipoproteins are removed, which can be carriers for lipophilic molecules (e.g., amiodarone, carbamazepine, lovastatin, and simvastatin) [7]. Yamamoto et al. demonstrated significant removal of amlodipine and ticlopidine (both lipoprotein bound medications) after LA; in contrast, no changes occurred in doxazosin level after LA (doxazosin is not lipoprotein-bound drug) [8].

RBC Exchange Several medications are redistributed in red blood cells (e.g., tacrolimus, cyclosporine A, sirolimus). Therefore, their removal via PEX is inefficient and attempts have been made for correction of drug toxicity via RBC exchange. Though several reports have been published, indicating significant reduction of sirolimus and tacrolimus levels after RBC exchange, the papers are generally case-reports, requiring larger controlled trails on the topic [7]. In addition, RBC exchange may cause HLA sensitization in solid organ transplantation as a long-term complication.

Hemoadsorption (HA) The data for medication removal during hemoadsorption is limited. Though the method was used for the treatment of poisoning before, the level of evidence is low due to the use of different adsorption columns, heterogeneity of studies (in vitro, animal, and human studies), as well as heterogeneity of agents evaluated (antibiotics, immunosuppressive agents) and clinical scenarios (e.g., poisoning, sepsis; adults or children). Finally, the published human studies are small, often case reports, lacking control group; usually HA is combined with other purification techniques [9].

- Antibiotics: different studies demonstrated significant removal of vancomycin, linezolid, gentamicin, meropenem and imipenem by different HA columns (Jafron HA series®, Jafron Biomedical Co., Ltd., Zhuhai, China; Cytosorb ®, Cytosorbents, Princetown, USA). However, another adsorption device (Seraph 100®, ExThera Medical, USA) did not increase clearance of azythromycin, cefazolin, cefepime, linezolid, vancomycin, indicating significant difference between adsorbers.
- Antithrombotic/anticoagulant drugs: HA significantly adsorbed ticagrelor and rivaroxaban and demonstrated

decreased bleeding risk in different clinical studies (data only for Cytosorb®).

- Immunosuppressive agents: HA did not significantly remove prednisolone, basiliximab, tacrolimus, cyclosporine A, mycophenolate, everolimus, and methylprednisolone. The study was performed in animal models [10]. In a single case, report HA removed effectively methotrexate in acute lymphocytic leukemia. Due to the very limited data, further studies are needed.
- Other medications: effective HA removal was demonstrated in clozapine, carbamazepine, and lamotrigine. Additionally, significant removal was established for amlodipine and iohexol.

Evaluating Drug Therapy Prior to PEX Treatment

Preferably, drug should be applied after PEX. However, if medication application prior to the procedure is required, the following risk factors for PEX removal should be considered if no data for PEX-associated reduction exists [3]:

- High protein binding (higher than 80%).
- Low Vd (lower than 0.2 L/kg).
- Longer half-life (more than 2 h).
- Drug application shortly prior to PEX.
- Presence of organ dysfunction, impairing drug elimination.
- Consider clinical importance of changes in drug concentrations.
- In unclear cases, therapeutic drug monitoring may guide drug dosing in PEX (e.g., aminoglycosides, vancomycin, antiepileptic drugs).

Removal of Specific Medications

Antimicrobials

Based on the small number of clinical trials and theoretical evaluation of antimicrobial pharmacokinetics, the following data on their PEX removal can be summarized [3, 11]:

- Significant removal: ceftriaxone, amphotericin B.
- Possible removal: ampicillin, amoxicillin, cefuroxime, vancomycin, aminoglycosides.
- Insignificant removal: carbapenems, fluconazole, voriconazole, acyclovir, fluoroquinolones, ganciclovir.

Immunosuppressive Agents

Similarly to antimicrobials, the data for the influence of PEX on immunosuppressive agents are limited. Their pharmacokinetics influences their PEX removal (e.g., Calcineurin inhibitors redistribute in RBC; biological agents have long half-lives and low *Vd*).

- Insignificant removal: Prednisolone/prednisone, Tacrolimus, Cyclosporin A, Mycophenolic acid [12].
- Significant removal: IVIG, monoclonal antibody therapies (Rituximab, Basiliximab, Natalizumab). The medications should be applied after PEX. In Rituximab, a study demonstrated up to 54% drug removal 25–66 h after the procedure. However, this may have no impact on its biological effect, as other studies demonstrated effective CD19+ and CD20+ B-lymphocyte depletion and clinical improvement in patients, treated with RTX prior to PEX [13, 14].

Antineoplastic Agents

- Insignificant removal: Methotrexate [12].
- Significant removal: Vincristine, Cisplatin [3].

Antiepileptic Drugs

Most of antiepileptic drugs have long half-lives with variable protein binding; however, *Vd* is usually higher than 0.2 L/kg.

In cases of PEX, therapeutic drug monitoring may be used to guide medication dosing.

Please note that minor transient changes in drug levels may be clinically significant.

- Possible removal: phenytoin, carbamazepine, valproic acid, levetiracetam, topiramate [3].

Anticoagulants and Cardiovascular Drugs

- Insignificant removal: digoxin, amiodarone.
- Possible removal: Amlodipine, Carvedilol, Verapamil, Diltiazem. Aspirin, Warfarin.
- Significant removal: Heparin, Enoxaparin, Deltaparin, Rivaroxaban, Aixaban, Lepirudin [3, 12].

Table 11.1 summarizes the data for drug removal by PEX and other apheresis techniques [3, 7, 9, 11].